Healthy Habits, Happy Life: Your Roadmap to Wellness

JARREL E.

Contents

1

Chapter 1

Introduction

Allow me to extend my gratitude for your interest in "Healthy Habits, Happy Life: Your Roadmap to Wellness." As a book author dedicated to providing valuable insights, I am honored to introduce you to this profound work, which aims to guide you on a transformative journey towards a happier and healthier life.

In our modern, fast-paced world, the pursuit of wellness has become paramount. People across the globe are seeking ways to enhance their physical, mental, and emotional well-being. "Healthy Habits, Happy Life" is a comprehensive exploration of the principles and practices that can lead you to a state of true vitality and contentment.

This book is not a mere collection of tips or quick fixes. It is a meticulously crafted roadmap, designed to empower you with the knowledge and tools needed to cultivate lasting, positive changes in your life. Drawing from the latest scientific research, time-tested wisdom, and practical strategies, "Healthy Habits, Happy Life" offers a holistic approach to well-being that addresses every facet of your existence.

Throughout the pages of this book, you will discover:

- **The Foundations of Wellness:** We will delve into the fundamental elements of well-being, including nutrition, exercise, sleep, and stress management. You will gain a deep understanding of how these factors interconnect and impact your overall health.
- **Mind-Body Harmony:** Explore the profound connection between your mental and physical health. Discover mindfulness techniques, stress reduction methods, and strategies for enhancing emotional resilience.
- **Nutritional Wisdom:** Uncover the secrets of a balanced diet and how it can energize your body, boost your immune system, and improve your mood. Learn how to make informed food choices that support your well-being.
- **The Power of Habits:** Dive into the science of habit formation and how to create sustainable, healthy routines that effortlessly become a part of your daily life.
- **Finding Joy and Fulfillment:** Explore the importance of purpose, relationships, and self-care in achieving a life filled with meaning and happiness.
- **Overcoming Challenges:** Address common obstacles on your wellness journey, such as time constraints, motivation dips, and setbacks, with practical strategies for resilience and perseverance.

Healthy Habits, Happy Life is more than just a guide; it is a companion on your path to a brighter, more fulfilling future. Each chapter is meticulously crafted to provide you with actionable insights, supported by evidence-based research, to help you make informed choices.

I invite you to embark on this transformative journey with me. Together, we will explore the intricacies of well-being and empower you to take control of your health and happiness. Whether you are a seasoned wellness enthusiast or just beginning to explore this path, this book is your trusted companion, offering guidance, inspiration, and the keys to unlocking a life of vitality and joy.

Thank you for entrusting me with the privilege of being your guide on this profound journey. Your pursuit of a healthier, happier life starts here.

The Importance of Health Habits

In the pursuit of a healthier and more fulfilling life, it is imperative that we recognize and appreciate the profound significance of health habits. These habits are the foundational building blocks upon which our well-being is constructed, and they hold the power to shape the trajectory of our lives. In this discourse, we shall delve deeply into the importance of health habits, elucidating why they are the cornerstones of a thriving existence.

- **Physical Vitality:** The first and most apparent benefit of health habits is their direct impact on physical well-being. Regular exercise, balanced nutrition, and adequate sleep are the keystones of physical vitality. Engaging in these habits not only boosts energy levels but also enhances physical strength, flexibility, and endurance. A well-nourished body is better equipped to ward off illnesses and injuries, ensuring a longer, healthier life.

- **Mental Clarity and Resilience:** Our cognitive functions are intimately linked to our lifestyle choices. Engaging in brain-boosting habits such as mindfulness meditation, adequate sleep, and a balanced diet can sharpen our mental acuity, improve memory, and bolster emotional resilience. These habits enable us to navigate the challenges of daily life with greater ease and composure.

- **Emotional Well-Being:** Health habits have a profound impact on our emotional state. Regular physical activity, for instance, releases endorphins, which are known as "feel-good" hormones, promoting a positive mood and reducing stress and anxiety. Moreover, a balanced diet rich in essential nutrients can stabilize mood swings and prevent emotional fluctuations.

- **Longevity:** The adoption of health habits has been linked to an increased lifespan. By mitigating the risk factors associated with chronic diseases such as heart disease, diabetes, and certain cancers, these habits can significantly contribute to a longer, more vibrant life. Additionally, habits like regular medical check-ups and preventive healthcare measures can catch potential issues early, further promoting longevity.

- **Quality of Life:** Health habits enhance our overall quality of life by optimizing our physical and mental well-being. When we feel well, we are more likely to engage in activities we enjoy, maintain strong relationships, and pursue our passions. This, in turn, leads to a more fulfilling and satisfying existence.

- **Positive Influence:** Embracing health habits can have a ripple effect, positively impacting those around us. Our choices can inspire family members, friends, and colleagues to adopt healthier lifestyles, thus creating a healthier community and society as a whole.

- **Cost Savings:** Lastly, it is worth noting that health habits can also lead to significant financial benefits. By preventing chronic illnesses, reducing medical expenses, and improving overall productivity, these habits can result in substantial cost savings over the long term.

Health habits are not merely a collection of routine actions; they are the pillars upon which a robust, fulfilling life is built. Their importance extends beyond the individual to the broader community and society, as the benefits of healthy living have far-reaching implications. It is incumbent upon each of us to recognize the paramount significance of health habits and take deliberate steps to incorporate them into our daily lives. By doing so, we unlock the potential for a brighter, more vital, and profoundly gratifying future.

How This Book Can Help You

Allow me to elucidate how the pages of this book can be a transformative force in your life. "Your Wellness Journey" is more than a mere collection of words; it is a comprehensive guide that has been meticulously crafted to empower you on your quest for a healthier, happier existence. Herein, we shall explore how this book can be your steadfast companion in achieving your wellness goals.

- **Knowledge and Understanding:** This book serves as a wellspring of knowledge, drawing from the latest scientific research, ancient wisdom, and practical insights. It provides a comprehensive understanding of the principles and practices that underpin well-being. By immersing yourself in its pages, you will gain a profound grasp of the factors that influence your health and happiness.
- **Actionable Insights:** Knowledge alone is insufficient; it is the application of that knowledge that yields results. "Your Wellness Journey" offers actionable insights, equipping you with practical strategies to implement in your daily life. Each chapter is replete with tips, techniques, and step-by-step guidance to help you create meaningful change.
- **Personalized Approach:** Recognizing that each individual is unique, this book offers a personalized approach to wellness. It encourages you to tailor the strategies to your specific needs, preferences, and circumstances. Whether you are a novice or an experienced wellness enthusiast, you will find guidance that suits your journey.
- **Holistic Perspective:** Wellness is not a singular facet but a holistic concept that encompasses physical, mental, and emotional well-being. This book takes a comprehensive view, addressing all these aspects, and emphasizes the interconnectedness of your health. It provides a roadmap for achieving balance and harmony in your life.
- **Motivation and Inspiration:** Embarking on a wellness journey can be challenging, and motivation can wane. "Your Wellness Journey" serves as a constant source of motivation and inspiration. It offers stories of real-life

individuals who have transformed their lives through these principles, showing you that change is not only possible but also attainable.

- **Overcoming Obstacles:** The path to wellness is not without its hurdles. This book recognizes common obstacles and provides strategies for overcoming them. Whether it's time constraints, motivation dips, or setbacks, you will find guidance on how to navigate these challenges with resilience.
- **Sustainable Habits:** One of the primary goals of this book is to help you cultivate sustainable, healthy habits. It delves into the science of habit formation, offering insights into how to make positive changes that endure over time. By the book's conclusion, you will be equipped with the tools to transform these habits into an integral part of your life.
- **Community and Support:** "Your Wellness Journey" fosters a sense of community and support. It encourages you to engage with others on similar journeys, whether through group activities, forums, or support networks. Knowing that you are not alone in your pursuit of well-being can be a powerful motivator.

This book is a dynamic companion on your journey to a healthier, happier life. It provides you with the knowledge, strategies, and motivation needed to embark on this transformative path. As you turn its pages and absorb its wisdom, remember that the power to change and thrive lies within you, and this book is your guide to unlock that potential.

Setting the Foundation

Before we delve into the intricacies of wellness, it is paramount that we begin by setting a solid foundation upon which our journey shall rest. The initial steps of any transformative endeavor are pivotal, for they lay the groundwork for the path ahead. In this chapter, we shall explore the essential elements that constitute this foundation, ensuring that you are well-prepared to embark on your wellness journey with clarity and purpose.

- **Clarity of Purpose:** Every meaningful journey begins with a clear sense of purpose. Take a moment to reflect upon why you are embarking on this wellness journey. Is it to improve your physical health, enhance your mental clarity, or find emotional balance? Is it to live a longer, more fulfilling life or to become a source of inspiration for your loved ones? Your purpose will serve as a guiding light, motivating you through challenges and setbacks.
- **Self-Reflection:** Self-awareness is a cornerstone of personal growth. Take time to reflect upon your current state of well-being. What areas of your life are thriving, and where do you perceive imbalances or challenges? Identifying these areas will help you set specific goals and priorities for your journey.
- **Goal Setting:** Setting clear, achievable goals is paramount to progress. Establish both short-term and long-term wellness goals that align with your purpose. These goals should be specific, measurable, and realistic. Whether it's adopting a regular exercise routine, improving your dietary choices, or enhancing your mental resilience, your goals will serve as the milestones on your path to success.
- **Education and Awareness:** Knowledge is a powerful tool

on the journey to wellness. Invest in your education about health and well-being. Familiarize yourself with the latest research, reputable resources, and expert advice. This knowledge will empower you to make informed decisions and choices.

- **Support Network:** Building a support network can be instrumental in your success. Share your wellness goals with friends, family, or peers who can offer encouragement and accountability. Seek out mentors, health professionals, or wellness communities that align with your objectives. Surrounding yourself with positive influences can greatly enhance your journey.
- **Mindset and Positivity:** Cultivate a positive mindset. Approach your wellness journey with an attitude of curiosity and self-compassion. Understand that setbacks are a natural part of growth, and each challenge is an opportunity to learn and adapt. A positive mindset will sustain your motivation and resilience.
- **Commitment:** Commitment to your well-being is non-negotiable. It requires dedication, consistency, and a willingness to prioritize your health. Be prepared to invest time and effort in your journey, recognizing that the benefits far outweigh the costs.
- **Flexibility and Adaptability:** Life is dynamic, and circumstances change. Flexibility and adaptability are essential qualities to cultivate. Understand that your wellness journey may need adjustments along the way. Embrace change as an opportunity for growth rather than a hindrance.

As you set this solid foundation, remember that you are embarking on a journey of self-discovery and transformation. The steps you take today will pave the way for a future filled with vitality, happiness, and fulfillment. With clarity of purpose, self-awareness, and unwavering commitment, you are well-prepared to take your first steps on this path toward a healthier, happier life.

Understanding Wellness

Before we embark on our profound journey towards well-being, it is essential that we establish a comprehensive understanding of what wellness truly entails. Wellness is not merely the absence of illness; it is a multifaceted state of thriving in every aspect of our lives. In this chapter, we shall delve deeply into the concept of wellness, exploring its various dimensions and how it pertains to our physical, mental, and emotional health.

Physical Wellness: At the core of wellness lies physical well-being. It encompasses the health of our bodies and our ability to maintain balance and vitality. Physical wellness encompasses:

- **Nutrition:** Consuming a balanced diet rich in essential nutrients that nourish our bodies and support optimal functioning.
- **Physical Activity:** Engaging in regular exercise to improve cardiovascular health, strength, flexibility, and endurance.
- **Rest and Recovery:** Ensuring adequate sleep and relaxation to allow our bodies to repair and rejuvenate.

Mental Wellness: Mental wellness pertains to the health of our cognitive and emotional faculties. It involves cultivating mental clarity, emotional resilience, and a positive outlook. Key aspects of mental wellness include:

- **Mindfulness:** Developing the ability to be fully present in the moment, reducing stress and enhancing self-awareness.
- **Emotional Intelligence:** Recognizing and managing our emotions effectively, fostering healthy relationships, and enhancing overall well-being.
- **Stress Management:** Implementing strategies to cope with stress, as chronic stress can have adverse effects on mental health.

Emotional Wellness: Emotional wellness revolves around our ability to navigate our emotions and maintain emotional balance. It involves:

- **Emotional Resilience:** Building the capacity to bounce back from challenges and setbacks with grace and adaptability.
- **Positive Relationships:** Cultivating healthy, supportive connections with others, which contribute significantly to emotional well-being.
- **Self-Compassion:** Treating ourselves with kindness and understanding, particularly during difficult times.

Social Wellness: Social wellness encompasses our interactions with others and our sense of belonging. It includes:

- **Community Engagement:** Participating in social activities, volunteering, or contributing to causes that align with our values.
- **Communication Skills:** Developing effective communica-

tion and conflict resolution skills to foster positive relation-ships.

- **Support Systems:** Building and nurturing a network of friends and family who provide emotional support and connection.

Spiritual Wellness: Spiritual wellness pertains to our sense of purpose and connection to something greater than ourselves. It includes:

- **Meaning and Purpose:** Finding meaning in life and align-ing our actions with our values and beliefs.
- **Meditation and Reflection:** Engaging in practices that promote inner peace, self-awareness, and a sense of tran-scendence.
- **Gratitude:** Cultivating an attitude of gratitude and appreci-ation for the present moment and life's blessings.

Environmental Wellness: Our well-being is also influenced by our environment. Environmental wellness involves:

- **Sustainable Living:** Making choices that minimize our impact on the environment and promote ecological balance.
- **Healthy Surroundings:** Ensuring that our living and work-ing spaces support our well-being, both physically and mentally.

In essence, wellness is a harmonious integration of these dimensions, and achieving it requires a balanced and holistic approach. It is not a destination but a lifelong journey that demands our attention and commitment. Understanding these

facets of wellness sets the stage for a comprehensive exploration of how to cultivate and maintain well-being in each area
of our lives.

As we continue on this journey together, I encourage you to
reflect on how each dimension of wellness resonates with your
own life. Recognize that wellness is a dynamic and evolving
concept, and your path may take unexpected turns. With a deep
understanding of wellness as our guide, we are well-equipped
to embark on this transformative journey.

Assessing Your Current Health

A crucial step in your journey toward well-being is an honest
assessment of your current health. To chart a path to a healthier,
happier life, it is essential to understand where you currently
stand in terms of your physical, mental, and emotional well-
being. In this chapter, we shall explore the process of assessing
your current health, providing you with the clarity needed to
make informed decisions and set meaningful goals.

Physical Health Assessment:

- **Medical Check-up:** Begin by scheduling a comprehensive
  medical check-up with your healthcare provider. This
  evaluation will include measurements of vital signs (e.g.,
  blood pressure, heart rate), blood tests, and an overall
  assessment of your physical health. Be sure to share any
  concerns or symptoms you may have.
- **Fitness Level:** Evaluate your current fitness level. Consider
  factors such as your cardiovascular endurance, strength,

flexibility, and body composition. You can perform simple fitness tests or consult with a fitness professional for a more in-depth assessment.

· **Nutrition Analysis:** Reflect on your dietary habits. Keep a food diary for a few days to gain insight into your eating patterns. Note whether your diet is rich in essential nutrients, or if it tends to be high in processed foods, sugars, or unhealthy fats.

· **Sleep Patterns:** Assess your sleep patterns. Reflect on the quality and duration of your sleep. Do you consistently get enough restful sleep, or do you struggle with insomnia or disrupted sleep?

Mental Health Assessment:

· **Stress Levels:** Reflect on your stress levels. Are you frequently overwhelmed, anxious, or experiencing chronic stress? Note any specific stressors in your life.

· **Mood and Emotions:** Consider your mood and emotional well-being. Are you generally content and positive, or do you often experience mood swings, sadness, or irritability? Pay attention to the frequency and intensity of these emotions.

· **Mindfulness and Presence:** Reflect on your ability to be present and mindful. Do you find yourself constantly distracted or preoccupied with worries and concerns? Assess your capacity to stay in the present moment.

Emotional Health Assessment:

· **Emotional Resilience:** Evaluate your emotional resilience.

How well do you cope with challenges, setbacks, and adversity? Are you able to bounce back from difficult experiences?

- **Interpersonal Relationships:** Consider the quality of your relationships with family, friends, and colleagues. Are these relationships supportive and fulfilling, or do they bring stress and negativity into your life?
- **Self-Care Practices:** Reflect on your self-care practices. Do you prioritize self-care activities that promote emotional well-being, such as relaxation, hobbies, or spending time in nature?

Lifestyle and Habits Assessment:

- **Habits:** Take an inventory of your daily habits, including diet, exercise, sleep, and relaxation. Identify which habits contribute positively to your well-being and which may be detrimental.
- **Substance Use:** Consider your use of substances such as alcohol, tobacco, or recreational drugs. Assess whether these substances have a significant impact on your health and well-being.
- **Environmental Factors:** Examine your living and working environment. Are there any environmental factors that may be affecting your health, such as air quality, noise, or stressors in your surroundings?

Remember that this assessment is not meant to be judgmental but rather a tool for self-awareness and reflection. It provides a baseline from which you can set realistic, meaningful goals for your wellness journey. It is essential to approach this process with self-compassion and a commitment to making positive changes that align with your vision of well-being.

As you reflect upon your current health, consider how each dimension of wellness we explored earlier contributes to your overall well-being. Your assessment will serve as a valuable reference point as we progress on this journey together, guiding you toward a brighter and healthier future.

Goal Setting for a Happier Life

One of the cornerstones of your journey toward a happier life is the art of setting meaningful and achievable goals. Goals serve as guiding stars, illuminating the path forward and motivating us to take purposeful actions. In this chapter, we shall delve into the profound process of goal setting, helping you craft objectives that resonate with your deepest desires and aspirations.

Clarity of Vision:

Begin by envisioning the life you aspire to lead. What does a happier life look like to you? Visualize the details: your relationships, career, physical health, emotional well-being, and personal growth. A clear vision forms the foundation of your goals.

SMART Goals:
Utilize the SMART criteria to structure your goals effectively:

- **Specific:** Define your goals with precision. Rather than a vague aim like "be healthier," specify "exercise for 30 minutes, five days a week" or "consume five servings of vegetables daily."

- **Measurable:** Your goals should be quantifiable. This enables you to track progress and measure success. For instance, instead of "improve fitness," opt for "run a 5K race in six months."
- **Achievable:** Ensure your goals are realistic and attainable. While it's admirable to aim high, set objectives that are within your reach, given your current circumstances and resources.
- **Relevant:** Your goals should align with your vision and values. They should be meaningful to you and contribute to your overall happiness and well-being.
- **Time-Bound:** Establish a timeframe for your goals. This creates a sense of urgency and commitment. For instance, "lose 10 pounds in three months" is time-bound.

Prioritization:

It's common to have numerous goals, but attempting to pursue all simultaneously can be overwhelming. Prioritize your goals by considering which are most pressing and align with your long-term vision. Focus on a manageable number at a time.

Break Down Larger Goals:

For ambitious long-term goals, break them down into smaller, actionable steps. This not only makes them less daunting but also provides a clear roadmap for progress. For example, if your goal is to write a book, break it down into daily or weekly writing targets.

Set Both Short-Term and Long-Term Goals:

While long-term goals provide a sense of direction, short-term goals offer milestones that keep you motivated and engaged. Balance your goal-setting by including objectives for the near future and those that span over time.

Regular Review:

Continuously assess your progress. Regularly reviewing your goals allows you to make adjustments, celebrate achievements, and stay accountable. Consider setting aside specific times for reflection, such as weekly or monthly check-ins.

Adaptability:

Life is dynamic, and circumstances change. Be open to adjusting your goals as needed. If unforeseen challenges arise or you discover new passions and interests, it's perfectly acceptable to modify your goals accordingly.

Stay Inspired:

Maintain your enthusiasm by keeping your vision and reasons for pursuing these goals at the forefront of your mind. Remind yourself why these objectives are essential for your happiness and well-being.

Seek Support and Accountability:

Share your goals with a trusted friend, mentor, or coach. Having someone to encourage you and hold you accountable can significantly boost your chances of success.

Practice Patience and Self-Compassion:

Achieving meaningful goals often takes time and effort. Embrace the journey with patience and self-compassion. Acknowledge that setbacks are part of growth, and use them as opportunities to learn and refine your approach.

In setting these goals for a happier life, remember that the pursuit of happiness is a journey, not a destination. Your goals are the milestones along this path, guiding you toward a life filled with fulfillment and contentment. With clarity, determination, and a steadfast commitment to your well-being, you are well-prepared to embark on this transformative journey.

2

Chapter 2

Nutrition for Vitality

As we continue our journey towards a happier and healthier life, one of the fundamental aspects we must address is nutrition. The food we consume is the fuel that powers our bodies and minds, and making wise nutritional choices is pivotal for vitality and well-being. In this chapter, we shall explore the principles of nutrition that promote vitality and energy.

Balanced Diet:

The cornerstone of optimal nutrition is a balanced diet that provides the body with a wide range of essential nutrients. Aim to include a variety of foods from all food groups:

- **Fruits and Vegetables:** Rich in vitamins, minerals, and antioxidants, fruits and vegetables are vital for overall health. Strive for a rainbow of colors to ensure diversity of nutrients.

- **Protein:** Incorporate lean protein sources such as poultry, fish, legumes, tofu, and nuts. Protein is crucial for muscle maintenance, immune function, and satiety.
- **Whole Grains:** Choose whole grains like brown rice, quinoa, whole wheat, and oats over refined grains. They provide sustained energy and fiber for digestive health.
- **Healthy Fats:** Include sources of healthy fats such as avocados, nuts, seeds, and olive oil. These fats support brain health and aid in the absorption of fat-soluble vitamins.
- **Dairy or Alternatives:** Opt for low-fat or non-dairy alternatives like almond milk or soy yogurt if you're lactose intolerant. Dairy products provide calcium and protein.

Portion Control:

While the quality of food is essential, portion control is equally important. Be mindful of portion sizes to avoid overeating. Pay attention to your body's hunger and fullness cues, and avoid eating to the point of discomfort.

Hydration:

Staying well-hydrated is vital for vitality. Water is essential for digestion, circulation, temperature regulation, and overall health. Aim to drink adequate water throughout the day, and consider herbal teas or infused water for variety.

Meal Timing:

Distribute your meals evenly throughout the day to maintain steady energy levels. Include breakfast to kickstart your metabolism, and avoid heavy, late-night meals that may disrupt sleep.

Mindful Eating:

Practice mindful eating by savoring each bite and paying attention to your body's hunger and fullness signals. Avoid distractions like screens or work during meals, and focus on the sensory experience of eating.

Limit Processed Foods:

Highly processed foods often contain excess sugar, salt, unhealthy fats, and additives. Minimize their consumption, and opt for whole, unprocessed foods whenever possible.

Moderation, Not Deprivation:

Wellness is about balance, not deprivation. Allow yourself occasional treats or indulgences while maintaining an overall nutritious diet. Enjoyment of food is an important aspect of well-being.

Customization:

Nutrition is not one-size-fits-all. Consider individual factors such as age, activity level, dietary preferences, and any specific health conditions when tailoring your diet to your unique needs.

Consult with Professionals:

If you have specific dietary concerns or health conditions, consider seeking guidance from a registered dietitian or health-care professional. They can provide personalized advice and support.

Lifelong Approach:

Remember that nutrition is a lifelong commitment to health and vitality. Sustainable changes over time are more effective than quick-fix diets. Aim for gradual, lasting improvements.

By embracing these principles of nutrition, you lay the foundation for increased vitality and energy in your daily life. Nutrient-rich foods support your physical and mental well-being, providing the sustained energy needed to pursue your goals and experience a happier, healthier life.

The Role of Nutrition in Wellness

In our pursuit of holistic well-being, the role of nutrition is undeniably central. Nutrition is not merely about satisfying our hunger; it is about providing our bodies with the essential nutrients required for optimal functioning, energy, and vitality. In this chapter, we shall explore in-depth the profound role that nutrition plays in our overall wellness.

Fuel for the Body:

Nutrition serves as the primary source of fuel for our bodies. The foods we consume are broken down into nutrients— carbohydrates, proteins, and fats— which provide energy for daily activities and bodily functions. A well-balanced diet ensures that we have the energy required for physical and mental tasks, supporting our overall well-being.

Nutrient Density:

Nutrient-dense foods provide a high concentration of essential nutrients relative to their calorie content. Fruits, vegetables, whole grains, lean proteins, and healthy fats are examples of nutrient-dense foods. These choices not only provide energy but also supply vitamins, minerals, and antioxidants that are crucial for health and vitality.

Immune System Support:

Proper nutrition is integral to a robust immune system. Nutrients such as vitamins C, D, and zinc, found in foods like citrus fruits, dairy products, and nuts, play a pivotal role in immune function. A well-nourished body is better equipped to fend off illnesses and infections.

Cellular Repair and Growth:

Proteins, obtained from sources like lean meats, fish, and legumes, are essential for the growth, repair, and maintenance of cells and tissues. They support muscle development, tissue healing, and overall structural integrity.

Brain Health:

Nutrition directly impacts cognitive function and mental well-being. Omega-3 fatty acids, found in fatty fish like salmon, support brain health and may improve mood. Antioxidants from fruits and vegetables help protect brain cells from oxidative stress.

Heart Health:

A heart-healthy diet, rich in fiber, healthy fats, and whole grains, can lower the risk of cardiovascular diseases. Foods like oats, olive oil, and nuts contribute to lower cholesterol levels and improved heart function.

Digestive Health:

Fiber, present in foods like whole grains, fruits, and vegetables, is essential for digestive health. It aids in regular bowel movements, prevents constipation, and supports a healthy gut microbiome.

Energy Balance:

Proper nutrition plays a pivotal role in achieving and maintaining a healthy weight. By consuming an appropriate balance of calories and nutrients, you can manage your weight effectively, reducing the risk of obesity-related health issues.

Mood and Emotional Well-Being:

The foods we eat can impact our mood and emotional well-being. Balanced meals that stabilize blood sugar levels can help regulate mood swings and prevent irritability. Additionally, certain nutrients, such as tryptophan found in turkey, can promote the production of serotonin, a neurotransmitter associated with feelings of happiness and well-being.

Longevity and Disease Prevention:

A nutritious diet is linked to longevity and the prevention of chronic diseases such as diabetes, heart disease, and certain cancers. Consistently making healthy food choices can significantly reduce the risk of these conditions.

Personalized Nutrition:

Recognize that individual nutrition needs can vary. Factors such as age, gender, activity level, and any specific health conditions must be considered when tailoring your diet to your unique requirements.

Lifestyle Integration:

Optimal nutrition is not an isolated aspect of wellness but an integral part of a broader lifestyle. Combining nutrition with other wellness practices, such as regular physical activity, mindfulness, and stress management, maximizes its impact on your overall well-being.

By understanding and embracing the role of nutrition in wellness, you empower yourself to make informed choices that positively influence your health and vitality. Nutrition is a cornerstone of well-being, and its profound impact extends to every facet of your life. It is an essential component of your wellness journey, one that can lead to a life filled with energy, vitality, and contentment.

Building a Balanced Diet

In the pursuit of a well-rounded and nourishing diet, it is imperative to build a balanced eating plan that provides your body with the essential nutrients it needs for vitality and well-being. A balanced diet is not about deprivation or strict rules; it is about making thoughtful choices that support your health. In this chapter, we shall explore the key principles for constructing a balanced diet.

Diverse Food Groups:

A balanced diet encompasses a variety of food groups, ensuring that your body receives a wide range of essential nutrients. The major food groups include:

Fruits and Vegetables: These are rich in vitamins, minerals, fiber, and antioxidants. Aim to fill half your plate with colorful fruits and vegetables at each meal.

Proteins: Lean proteins from sources like poultry, fish, lean cuts of meat, legumes, tofu, and nuts provide essential amino acids for muscle repair and overall health.

Whole Grains: Whole grains like brown rice, quinoa, whole wheat pasta, and oats offer complex carbohydrates, fiber, vitamins, and minerals for sustained energy.

Healthy Fats: Include sources of healthy fats such as avocados, nuts, seeds, and olive oil. These fats support brain health and overall well-being.

Dairy or Alternatives: Dairy products provide calcium and protein. If you are lactose intolerant, consider non-dairy alternatives like almond milk or soy yogurt.

Portion Control:

While the quality of food is crucial, portion control is equally important. Be mindful of portion sizes to avoid overeating. Listen to your body's hunger and fullness cues.

Moderation and Balance:

A balanced diet includes all food groups in moderation. Avoid excessive consumption of any single type of food, as this can lead to nutritional imbalances.

Color and Diversity:

Aim to eat a colorful and diverse range of foods. Different colors in fruits and vegetables signify various nutrients and antioxidants. A diverse diet ensures a wide array of nutrients.

Lean Protein Sources:

Opt for lean protein sources to reduce saturated fat intake. Poultry, fish, legumes, and tofu are excellent choices for protein without excessive fat.

Whole Grains:

Choose whole grains over refined grains. Whole grains are rich in fiber, vitamins, and minerals. They provide sustained energy and support digestive health.

Healthy Fats:

Incorporate healthy fats in your diet. Avocados, nuts, seeds, and olive oil contain monounsaturated and polyunsaturated fats, which promote heart and brain health.

Limit Processed Foods:

Highly processed foods often contain excess sugar, salt, unhealthy fats, and additives. Minimize their consumption and opt for whole, unprocessed foods.

Hydration:

Don't forget the importance of staying well-hydrated. Water is essential for digestion, circulation, temperature regulation, and overall health. Aim to drink adequate water throughout the day.

Mindful Eating:

Practice mindful eating by savoring each bite and paying attention to your body's hunger and fullness signals. Avoid distractions like screens during meals.

Personalized Approach:

Customize your diet to your individual needs and preferences. Consider factors such as age, activity level, dietary restrictions, and any specific health conditions.

Balanced Lifestyle:

Remember that a balanced diet is just one facet of a holistic wellness plan. Complement your nutrition with regular physical activity, stress management, and adequate sleep.

By adhering to these principles, you create a balanced diet that not only nourishes your body but also supports your overall well-being. A balanced diet is not about rigid rules but about cultivating a sustainable and enjoyable approach to eating. It is a key component of your wellness journey, one that leads to a life filled with energy, vitality, and health.

Mindful Eating Practices

Mindful eating is a practice that can profoundly transform your relationship with food, enhance your overall well-being, and promote a healthier and happier life. In this chapter, we shall explore the art of mindful eating and the principles that can guide you toward a more conscious and satisfying approach to nourishing your body.

Presence and Awareness:

Mindful eating begins with being fully present in the moment.

When you sit down to eat, eliminate distractions such as television, smartphones, or work. Focus your attention solely on the meal in front of you.

Engage Your Senses:

Use your senses to fully experience your food. Notice the colors, textures, and aromas of your meal. Take small, deliberate bites, and savor each one. Chew slowly and savor the flavors as they unfold on your palate.

Listen to Your Body:

Pay attention to your body's hunger and fullness cues. Before you begin eating, assess your level of hunger. Are you eating out of true hunger, or is it due to boredom, stress, or habit? During the meal, pause periodically to check in with your body's signals of fullness.

Observe Emotional Eating:

Be mindful of emotional eating patterns. Notice if you turn to food as a way to cope with stress, sadness, or boredom. When you are aware of these patterns, you can make more conscious choices about how to address your emotions without relying on food.

Appreciation and Gratitude:

Cultivate an attitude of appreciation and gratitude for the nourishment your meal provides. Reflect on the journey the food took to reach your plate, from the farmers who grew it to the hands that prepared it. This perspective can deepen your connection to your food.

Eat with Intention:

Set an intention for your meal. Consider what you hope to gain from this nourishing experience. Whether it's energy for your day, nourishment for your body, or simply enjoyment, having an intention can guide your eating choices.

Portion Awareness:

Be mindful of portion sizes. Use smaller plates and serving utensils to help control portion sizes. This can prevent overeating and encourage you to savor each bite.

No Judgment:

Approach your meal without judgment. There are no "good" or "bad" foods. Release any guilt or shame associated with eating. Instead, focus on the nourishment and enjoyment that your food provides.

Mindful Meal Planning:

Extend mindfulness to meal planning and preparation. Select foods that align with your well-being goals, and take the time to prepare meals with care and attention.

Practice Mindful Eating Regularly:

Mindful eating is a practice that deepens with regularity. Incorporate it into your daily routine, starting with one meal or snack each day. Gradually, you can expand this practice to more of your eating occasions.

Reflect and Learn:

After your mindful meal, take a moment to reflect on the experience. What did you notice about your eating habits, thoughts, and sensations? Use this self-awareness to make conscious choices in future meals.

By embracing mindful eating practices, you can transform your relationship with food and your overall well-being. It allows you to savor the joy of eating, make more conscious choices, and develop a healthier and more satisfying approach to nourishing your body and soul. Mindful eating is a valuable tool on your wellness journey, one that can lead to a happier and more balanced life.

3

Chapter 3

The Power of Physical Activity

Physical activity is a powerful catalyst for vitality, well-being, and overall health. It has the potential to transform your life by enhancing physical fitness, boosting mental and emotional well-being, and contributing to a happier and healthier existence. In this chapter, we shall explore the profound power of physical activity and how it can positively impact your journey toward wellness.

Physical Fitness:

Engaging in regular physical activity is fundamental to building and maintaining physical fitness. It enhances cardiovascular health, increases muscular strength and endurance, improves flexibility, and promotes a healthy body composition. Physical fitness not only enhances your physical capabilities but also contributes to your overall well-being.

Mental Clarity and Cognitive Function:

Physical activity has a remarkable impact on mental clarity and cognitive function. Regular exercise increases blood flow to the brain, which can enhance memory, concentration, and cognitive abilities. It also stimulates the release of neurotransmitters like endorphins, which contribute to a positive mood and reduced stress.

Emotional Well-Being:

Physical activity is a powerful mood enhancer. It can alleviate symptoms of depression and anxiety by releasing feel-good chemicals like serotonin and reducing the levels of stress hormones. Regular exercise also provides a sense of accomplishment and self-confidence, fostering emotional well-being.

Stress Reduction:

Physical activity is a natural stress reliever. It helps the body and mind cope with stress by reducing the production of stress hormones and promoting relaxation. Engaging in physical activity, such as yoga or mindfulness-based exercises, can be particularly effective for stress management.

Weight Management:

Regular physical activity plays a pivotal role in weight management. It helps burn calories and build lean muscle, which can contribute to maintaining a healthy weight. It also supports metabolic health, making it easier to manage body weight.

Cardiovascular Health:

Aerobic exercises like walking, running, swimming, and cycling are excellent for cardiovascular health. They strengthen the heart, lower blood pressure, and improve circulation, reducing the risk of heart disease.

Bone Health:

Weight-bearing exercises, such as resistance training and weightlifting, are essential for bone health. They help build and maintain bone density, reducing the risk of osteoporosis and fractures.

Improved Sleep:

Regular physical activity can lead to improved sleep quality. It helps regulate sleep patterns and promotes deeper, more restful sleep, which is vital for overall well-being.

Enhanced Longevity:

Research consistently shows that individuals who engage in regular physical activity tend to live longer, healthier lives. Physical activity reduces the risk of chronic diseases and contributes to a longer, more active lifespan.

Lifestyle Integration:

Incorporate physical activity into your daily life to maximize its benefits. This can include walking or biking to work, taking the stairs instead of the elevator, or engaging in recreational activities you enjoy.

Personalized Approach:

Recognize that the type and intensity of physical activity should align with your individual preferences, fitness level, and any specific health conditions. Consult with a healthcare professional if needed.

By harnessing the power of physical activity, you take significant steps toward a life filled with vitality, energy, and happiness. Whether it's through structured exercise routines, outdoor activities, or simply incorporating more movement into your daily life, physical activity is a cornerstone of your wellness journey.

Benefits of Regular Exercise

Regular exercise is a potent elixir for a happier, healthier life. It bestows a multitude of benefits upon those who embrace it, enhancing physical fitness, mental well-being, and overall quality of life. In this chapter, we shall explore the manifold advantages of incorporating regular exercise into your wellness journey.

Improved Cardiovascular Health:

Engaging in regular exercise strengthens the heart and enhances cardiovascular health. It lowers the risk of heart disease by reducing levels of "bad" LDL cholesterol, improving blood pressure, and increasing overall circulation.

Enhanced Physical Fitness:

Regular physical activity improves physical fitness across various dimensions:

Endurance: Exercise increases your stamina, allowing you to engage in daily activities with less fatigue.

Strength: Resistance training builds muscle strength, supporting better posture and functionality.

Flexibility: Stretching exercises improve flexibility and range of motion, reducing the risk of injury.

Weight Management:

Exercise contributes to weight management by burning calories and building lean muscle mass. It aids in both weight loss and weight maintenance, making it easier to achieve and sustain a healthy body weight.

Mood Elevation:

Regular exercise is a natural mood enhancer. It stimulates the release of endorphins, which are often referred to as "feel-good" hormones. These endorphins promote a positive mood, reduce stress, and combat symptoms of depression and anxiety.

Stress Reduction:

Physical activity is a powerful stress reducer. It helps the body manage stress by reducing the production of stress hormones and promoting relaxation. Engaging in exercise can provide a sense of calm and emotional well-being.

Better Sleep:

Regular exercise can improve sleep quality. It regulates sleep patterns and promotes deeper, more restful sleep, which is essential for overall well-being and cognitive function.

Bone Health:

Weight-bearing exercises, such as resistance training and weightlifting, are essential for bone health. They help build and maintain bone density, reducing the risk of osteoporosis and fractures.

Enhanced Cognitive Function:

Exercise has a positive impact on cognitive function and brain health. It increases blood flow to the brain, which can enhance memory, concentration, and cognitive abilities.

Increased Energy Levels:

Engaging in regular physical activity boosts energy levels and combats fatigue. It can improve overall vitality and make daily tasks feel more manageable.

Longevity and Disease Prevention:

Research consistently shows that individuals who maintain a regular exercise regimen tend to live longer, healthier lives. Exercise reduces the risk of chronic diseases such as diabetes, heart disease, and certain cancers.

Improved Immune Function:

Regular exercise supports a healthy immune system. It can enhance the body's ability to defend against illnesses and infections.

Lifestyle Integration:

Incorporating physical activity into your daily life, such as walking or biking for transportation, gardening, or dancing, ensures a sustainable and enjoyable approach to exercise.

Personalized Approach:

Recognize that the type, duration, and intensity of exercise should align with your individual preferences, fitness level, and any specific health conditions. Consult with a healthcare professional if needed.

By embracing regular exercise, you unlock a wealth of physical and mental benefits that can lead to a life filled with vitality, happiness, and improved overall well-being. Exercise is a potent tool on your wellness journey, one that empowers you to live your best life.

Finding Your Fitness Passion

Discovering and embracing your fitness passion can be a transformative journey that enhances your overall well-being and joy in life. When you engage in physical activities that you love and are passionate about, exercise becomes an integral and enjoyable part of your daily routine. In this chapter, we shall explore the process of finding your fitness passion and reaping the benefits it brings to your wellness journey.

Self-Exploration:

Begin by exploring your interests and preferences. Reflect on the physical activities that have intrigued or excited you in the past. Consider the activities you enjoyed during childhood or any hobbies that involve movement.

Try a Variety of Activities:

To find your fitness passion, be open to trying a variety of physical activities. Attend different classes, join sports clubs, or experiment with solo pursuits. This exploration process allows you to discover what resonates with you.

Listen to Your Body:

Pay attention to how your body responds to different activities. Note the physical sensations, emotions, and sense of fulfillment you experience during and after each activity. Your body often provides valuable feedback about what resonates with you.

Consider Your Goals:

Think about your fitness and wellness goals. Are you interested in building strength, improving flexibility, enhancing cardiovascular fitness, or simply having fun? Align your chosen activities with your goals for a more purposeful approach.

Connect with Your Interests:

If you have specific interests outside of fitness, explore how they can be integrated into physical activities. For example, if you love nature, consider hiking or outdoor yoga. If you enjoy music, dance-based fitness classes might be appealing.

Explore Social Opportunities:

Many people find motivation and enjoyment in group fitness classes or team sports. Joining a fitness community or sports league can provide social connections and a sense of camaraderie.

Engage Your Creativity:

Some fitness activities allow for creative expression. Dance, martial arts, and various forms of yoga often incorporate artistic and expressive elements.

Assess Your Lifestyle:

Consider your daily routine and lifestyle. Some fitness activities may be more accessible and compatible with your schedule and location than others.

Set Realistic Expectations:

Understand that it may take time to discover your fitness passion. Be patient with yourself and allow the process to unfold naturally. What matters is that you're actively exploring and enjoying the journey.

Personalized Approach:

Remember that your fitness journey is highly personal. What brings passion and joy to one person may differ from another's experience. Embrace the activities that genuinely resonate with you.

Consistency Is Key:

Once you find your fitness passion, make it a consistent part of your routine. Regular engagement not only enhances your fitness but also deepens your connection to the activity.

Finding your fitness passion is an empowering step on your wellness journey. It transforms exercise from a chore into a source of joy and fulfillment. When you genuinely enjoy the physical activities you engage in, you're more likely to maintain a consistent fitness routine and reap the physical and mental benefits that come with it.

Creating a Sustainable Exercise Routine

Creating a sustainable exercise routine is key to achieving long-term fitness goals and maintaining a healthy lifestyle.

Sustainability ensures that exercise becomes a consistent and enjoyable part of your life, rather than a short-term effort. In this chapter, we shall explore the principles of building a sustainable exercise routine that aligns with your wellness journey.

Set Realistic Goals:

Start by setting realistic and achievable fitness goals. Whether it's improving cardiovascular health, building strength, or increasing flexibility, having clear and attainable objectives provides direction for your routine.

Choose Activities You Love:

Opt for physical activities that you genuinely enjoy. When you engage in exercises you love, it becomes easier to stay motivated and committed. Whether it's dancing, hiking, swimming, or team sports, find activities that resonate with you.

Variety and Diversity:

Incorporate a variety of exercises into your routine. This prevents boredom, reduces the risk of overuse injuries, and ensures that you work different muscle groups. Mix cardio, strength training, flexibility, and balance exercises for a well-rounded approach.

Prioritize Consistency Over Intensity:

Consistency is the foundation of a sustainable routine. It's better to engage in moderate-intensity exercise regularly than to push yourself to the extreme sporadically. Aim for a sustainable pace that you can maintain over time.

Set a Realistic Schedule:

Consider your daily life and obligations when setting your exercise schedule. Choose times that are convenient and realistic for you. Consistency is more important than the specific time of day you exercise.

Start Slowly:

If you're new to exercise or making a comeback, start slowly to avoid burnout or injury. Gradually increase the intensity and duration of your workouts as your fitness level improves.

Listen to Your Body:

Pay attention to your body's signals. If you feel fatigued, sore, or experience discomfort, it's okay to take a rest day or engage in lighter exercise. Pushing through pain can lead to injury and disrupt sustainability.

Rest and Recovery:

Adequate rest and recovery are essential for sustainability. Allow your body time to repair and rejuvenate between workouts. Include rest days in your routine and prioritize quality sleep.

Set Milestones, Not Deadlines:

Instead of focusing on achieving a specific fitness level by a certain date, set milestones along the way. Celebrate your progress and recognize that fitness is an ongoing journey, not a destination.

Incorporate Flexibility:

Be flexible with your routine. Life can be unpredictable, and there may be days when you can't follow your plan exactly. Adapt by finding alternative ways to stay active or reschedule your workouts.

Seek Support and Accountability:

Consider partnering with a workout buddy or joining a fitness group. Having support and accountability can boost motivation and make exercise more enjoyable.

Track Your Progress:

Keep a record of your workouts and progress. This allows you to see how far you've come and can be motivating. It also helps you identify areas for improvement.

Reevaluate and Adjust:

Periodically reassess your goals, routine, and fitness preferences. As your needs and interests evolve, adjust your exercise routine accordingly to keep it fresh and engaging.

Building a sustainable exercise routine is a crucial step on your wellness journey. It ensures that fitness becomes an integral and enjoyable part of your life, contributing to your physical and mental well-being over the long term. Remember that sustainability is about consistency, enjoyment, and adaptability.

4

Chapter 4

Rest and Sleep

Rest and sleep are pillars of wellness that play an indispensable role in your journey toward a happier and healthier life. Proper rest and sleep are essential for physical and mental rejuvenation, maintaining optimal cognitive function, and supporting overall well-being. In this chapter, we shall delve into the importance of rest and sleep and explore strategies to ensure you get the rejuvenating rest you need.

The Significance of Rest:

Physical Recovery:

Rest is crucial for the body's physical recovery. During rest, tissues repair, muscles rebuild, and energy stores are replenished. It is the body's way of healing and preparing for the challenges of the day ahead.

Mental Refreshment:

Mental rest is equally important. It allows the mind to recuperate from the demands of daily life, reducing mental fatigue and improving cognitive function. Mental rest can enhance creativity, problem-solving abilities, and overall productivity.

Stress Reduction:

Adequate rest is a potent stress reducer. It provides a break from the daily stressors of life and allows the body to regulate stress hormones, promoting emotional well-being.

Improved Concentration:

Restorative sleep and regular breaks during the day enhance concentration and focus. They help you stay alert, make better decisions, and perform tasks more efficiently.

Enhanced Physical Performance:

Athletes and fitness enthusiasts benefit from rest as it supports physical performance and recovery. It is during rest that muscles adapt and become stronger, making it an integral part of any training regimen.

The Importance of Sleep:

Physical Health:

Quality sleep is essential for physical health. It supports

immune function, hormone regulation, and cardiovascular health. Lack of sleep is associated with an increased risk of chronic diseases such as diabetes, obesity, and heart disease.

Mental Well-Being:

Sleep is a cornerstone of mental well-being. It contributes to emotional stability, mood regulation, and the prevention of mood disorders like depression and anxiety.

Cognitive Function:

Adequate sleep is vital for cognitive function. It consolidates memories, enhances problem-solving skills, and supports learning and creativity. Sleep deprivation can lead to cognitive deficits, impaired judgment, and decreased productivity.

Stress Management:

Sleep is an essential component of stress management. It helps regulate stress hormones, reduces the perception of stressors, and enhances resilience to life's challenges.

Weight Management:

Quality sleep is linked to weight management. It regulates hunger hormones, reducing the likelihood of overeating and weight gain.

Strategies for Rest and Sleep:

Prioritize Sleep: Set a consistent sleep schedule and aim for 7-9 hours of quality sleep each night.

Create a Relaxing Bedtime Routine: Develop pre-sleep rituals like reading, gentle stretching, or meditation to signal to your body that it's time to wind down.

Optimize Sleep Environment: Ensure your bedroom is conducive to sleep with a comfortable mattress, appropriate bedding, and a dark, quiet, and cool atmosphere.

Limit Screen Time: Reduce exposure to screens (phones, computers, TVs) before bedtime, as the blue light emitted can interfere with the production of the sleep hormone melatonin.

Regular Physical Activity: Engage in regular physical activity to promote better sleep. However, avoid strenuous exercise close to bedtime.

Mindful Rest Breaks: Take short, mindful breaks during the day to recharge. This can include deep breathing, stretching, or a brief walk.

Stress Management: Practice stress management techniques such as meditation, yoga, or journaling to reduce stress and promote relaxation.

Limit Caffeine and Alcohol: Avoid consuming caffeine and alcohol close to bedtime, as they can disrupt sleep patterns.

Consult a Healthcare Professional: If you experience persistent sleep difficulties or rest-related concerns, consult a healthcare professional for guidance and evaluation.

Rest and sleep are vital components of your wellness journey. Embrace them as essential practices that support your physical and mental well-being, and you will experience a profound improvement in the quality of your life.

Prioritizing Quality Sleep

Prioritizing quality sleep is a cornerstone of your wellness journey. Quality sleep rejuvenates your body and mind, enhancing physical and mental well-being, cognitive function, and overall vitality. In this chapter, we shall delve into strategies for prioritizing and optimizing the quality of your sleep for a happier and healthier life.

Creating a Sleep-Enhancing Environment:

Set a Consistent Sleep Schedule:

Go to bed and wake up at the same time every day, even on weekends. A regular sleep schedule helps regulate your body's internal clock.

Optimize Your Sleep Environment:

Ensure your bedroom is conducive to sleep. This includes a comfortable mattress and pillows, appropriate bedding, and a dark, quiet, and cool atmosphere.

Limit Exposure to Screens:

The blue light emitted by screens (phones, computers, TVs) can interfere with your sleep. Minimize screen time at least an hour before bedtime, or use blue light filters on your devices.

Create a Relaxing Bedtime Routine:

Develop pre-sleep rituals to signal to your body that it's time to wind down. Activities like reading, gentle stretching, or meditation can help relax your mind and prepare you for sleep.

Mindful Rest Breaks:

Take short, mindful breaks during the day to recharge. Deep breathing, stretching, or a brief walk can help reduce stress and enhance your overall sense of well-being.

Healthy Sleep Habits:

Limit Caffeine and Alcohol:

Avoid consuming caffeine and alcohol close to bedtime, as they can disrupt sleep patterns. Opt for caffeine-free herbal teas or warm milk instead.

Watch Your Diet:

Heavy or spicy meals before bedtime can cause discomfort and indigestion. It's advisable to finish eating at least 2-3 hours before sleep.

Stay Active, But Not Too Late:

Regular physical activity supports better sleep, but avoid strenuous exercise close to bedtime. Aim to finish exercise at least a few hours before sleep.

Limit Naps:

While short power naps can be refreshing, long or irregular daytime naps can interfere with nighttime sleep. If you nap, keep it brief (20-30 minutes) and early in the day.

Manage Stress:

Practice stress management techniques such as meditation, progressive muscle relaxation, or deep breathing exercises to reduce stress and promote relaxation before bedtime.

Prioritizing Your Sleep Needs:

Listen to Your Body:

Pay attention to your body's signals. If you're tired, allow yourself to rest or take a nap if possible. Ignoring fatigue can lead to sleep deprivation.

Create a Wind-Down Period:

Dedicate the hour before bedtime to calming activities that help you relax. This includes reading, taking a warm bath, or practicing relaxation exercises.

Limit Clock-Watching:

Constantly checking the time can create anxiety about not sleeping. If you can't sleep, try to stay relaxed and avoid looking at the clock.

Seek Professional Help:

If you consistently struggle with sleep or experience sleep disorders, consider consulting a healthcare professional or sleep specialist for guidance and evaluation.

Quality sleep is a precious asset on your wellness journey. By prioritizing and optimizing the quality of your sleep, you unlock a wealth of benefits for your physical and mental well-being, cognitive function, and overall quality of life. Approach sleep as a cherished practice that nurtures your body and mind, and you will reap the rewards of a healthier and happier existence.

Stress Management Techniques

Stress management is a vital skill on your journey toward wellness and a happier, healthier life. In our fast-paced world, stress can accumulate and take a toll on both your physical and mental well-being. In this chapter, we shall explore a variety of stress management techniques that empower you to effectively cope with and reduce stress.

Mindfulness and Relaxation Techniques:

Mindfulness Meditation:

Mindfulness meditation involves paying focused attention to the present moment without judgment. Regular practice can enhance your ability to manage stress by promoting relaxation and reducing anxiety.

Deep Breathing Exercises:

Deep breathing exercises, such as diaphragmatic or abdominal breathing, can calm your nervous system and reduce stress. Practice these exercises during moments of tension or as part of a daily relaxation routine.

Progressive Muscle Relaxation:

Progressive muscle relaxation involves tensing and then relaxing different muscle groups in your body. It promotes physical and mental relaxation, helping you release tension and stress.

Yoga and Tai Chi:

Yoga and Tai Chi are mind-body practices that combine physical postures with breath control and meditation. They promote relaxation, flexibility, and stress reduction.

Lifestyle and Wellness Practices:

Regular Physical Activity:

Engaging in regular exercise is a potent stress reducer. It releases endorphins, improves mood, and helps your body manage stress more effectively.

Healthy Diet:

Proper nutrition plays a significant role in stress management. A balanced diet that includes fruits, vegetables, whole grains, lean proteins, and healthy fats supports overall well-being.

Adequate Sleep:

Prioritize quality sleep to recharge your body and mind. Sleep is essential for stress recovery and emotional well-being.

Time Management:

Effective time management can reduce stress related to work or daily responsibilities. Organize your tasks, set priorities, and allocate time for relaxation and self-care.

Social Support:

Maintain strong social connections. Talking to friends, family, or a therapist can provide emotional support and help you navigate challenging situations.

Cognitive and Emotional Techniques:

Positive Self-Talk:

Practice positive self-talk by replacing negative or catastrophic thoughts with realistic and constructive ones. This can help reduce anxiety and improve your ability to cope with stressors.

Journaling:

Keeping a journal can be a therapeutic way to express your thoughts and emotions. It allows you to gain insight into your stressors and identify strategies for managing them.

Mindful Acceptance:

Embrace the practice of accepting things you cannot change. Focus on what you can control and let go of the rest. This can reduce stress associated with trying to control the uncontrollable.

Visualization:

Visualization techniques involve imagining a calm and peaceful place or scenario. Visualization can help you relax and reduce stress by taking your mind to a tranquil mental space.

Professional Guidance:

Therapy and Counseling:

Consider seeking the guidance of a therapist or counselor, especially if you're dealing with chronic stress or specific stressors. They can provide coping strategies and support.

Mind-Body Therapies:

Mind-body therapies such as acupuncture, massage therapy, or biofeedback can complement stress management efforts and promote relaxation.

Stress management is a skill that can be developed and refined over time. By integrating these techniques into your daily life and customizing them to your specific needs, you empower yourself to effectively manage stress and cultivate a sense of balance and well-being. Remember that stress is a natural part of life, but with the right tools, you can navigate it with grace and resilience.

Relaxation and Mindfulness

Relaxation and mindfulness are invaluable practices that promote inner calm, mental clarity, and overall well-being. In our fast-paced world, cultivating these practices is essential for reducing stress and enhancing your quality of life. In this chapter, we shall explore relaxation and mindfulness techniques that empower you to find tranquility amid life's demands.

Relaxation Techniques:

Deep Breathing Exercises:

Deep breathing exercises, such as diaphragmatic breathing, can quickly induce relaxation. Inhale deeply through your nose, allowing your abdomen to rise, then exhale slowly through your mouth, letting go of tension.

Progressive Muscle Relaxation:

Progressive muscle relaxation involves systematically tensing and then relaxing different muscle groups in your body. It promotes physical and mental relaxation, helping you release tension and stress.

Guided Imagery:

Guided imagery involves using your imagination to create a mental scene that promotes relaxation. Visualize a peaceful place or scenario, engaging all your senses to enhance the experience.

Body Scan Meditation:

Body scan meditation involves focusing your attention on each part of your body, starting from your toes and moving upward. It helps you become aware of physical sensations and release tension.

Autogenic Training:

Autogenic training uses self-suggestions to promote relaxation. It involves repeating phrases like "my arms are heavy and warm," which can induce a state of physical relaxation.

Mindfulness Practices:

Mindful Breathing:

Mindful breathing is a core mindfulness practice. Pay close attention to your breath as you inhale and exhale. If your mind wanders, gently bring your focus back to your breath.

Mindful Eating:

When eating, practice mindful eating by savoring each bite, paying attention to textures and flavors, and eating without distractions. This fosters a deeper connection with your food.

Body Scan Meditation:

As mentioned earlier, body scan meditation is a mindfulness practice that involves observing physical sensations in your body with non-judgmental awareness.

Mindful Walking:

Mindful walking is a practice of walking slowly and attentively, focusing on the sensations of each step and your connection with the earth beneath you.

Loving-Kindness Meditation:

Loving-kindness meditation involves generating feelings of love and compassion for yourself and others. It cultivates a sense of kindness and empathy in your daily interactions.

Incorporating Relaxation and Mindfulness Into Daily Life:

Start Small:

Begin with short, manageable sessions of relaxation or mindfulness. Gradually extend the duration as you become more comfortable with the practice.

Set Aside Time:

Dedicate specific times for relaxation or mindfulness each day. It can be in the morning, during breaks, or before bedtime. Consistency is key.

Create a Peaceful Space:

Find a quiet and comfortable space for your practice. It could be a cozy corner in your home, a park, or any place where you can focus without distractions.

Stay Present:

During your practice, gently bring your attention back to the present moment if your mind wanders. Be patient and non-judgmental with yourself.

Integrate Mindfulness Into Daily Activities:

Practice mindfulness during everyday activities like washing dishes, commuting, or waiting in line. Use these moments to stay present and cultivate mindfulness.

Relaxation and mindfulness are powerful tools for managing stress, enhancing mental clarity, and fostering emotional well-being. As you embrace these practices, you empower yourself to find tranquility and balance in the midst of life's challenges.

They are not merely techniques; they are gateways to a more peaceful and fulfilling existence.

$$5$$

Chapter 5

Mental and Emotional Well-Being

Mental and emotional well-being are pillars of your wellness journey, contributing significantly to your overall happiness and quality of life. In this chapter, we shall explore the importance of mental and emotional well-being and provide strategies to nurture and maintain them.

Understanding Mental and Emotional Well-Being:

Mental Well-Being:

Mental well-being encompasses your cognitive and emotional state. It involves having a positive sense of self, feeling capable of managing life's challenges, and maintaining mental resilience.

Emotional Well-Being:

Emotional well-being relates to your emotional state and how effectively you can manage and express your emotions. It involves experiencing a range of emotions in a healthy way and having the skills to cope with emotional challenges.

Strategies for Nurturing Mental and Emotional Well-Being:

Self-Awareness:

Cultivate self-awareness by regularly reflecting on your thoughts, feelings, and behaviors. Recognize and acknowledge your emotions, and identify any patterns that may affect your well-being.

Emotional Regulation:

Develop skills for managing and regulating your emotions. Techniques such as deep breathing, mindfulness, and journaling can help you understand and cope with your feelings effectively.

Positive Self-Talk:

Practice positive self-talk by challenging and reframing negative thoughts. Replace self-criticism with self-compassion and self-encouragement.

Healthy Coping Mechanisms:

Identify healthy ways to cope with stress and adversity. Engage in activities that bring you joy, such as hobbies, exercise, or spending time with loved ones.

Social Support:

Maintain strong social connections with friends and family. Sharing your thoughts and feelings with trusted individuals can provide emotional support and perspective.

Seek Professional Help:

If you're struggling with persistent mental or emotional challenges, consider seeking the guidance of a mental health professional. Therapy or counseling can provide valuable tools and strategies for improvement.

Stress Management:

Stress Awareness:

Be mindful of your stressors and their impact on your mental and emotional well-being. Identify sources of stress and their effects on your thoughts and emotions.

Stress Reduction Techniques:

Engage in stress-reduction techniques such as meditation, deep breathing exercises, and progressive muscle relaxation to alleviate stress and promote relaxation.

Healthy Lifestyle Habits:

Physical Activity:

Regular exercise is not only beneficial for physical health but also for mental and emotional well-being. It releases endorphins, reduces stress, and improves mood.

Nutrition:

Maintain a balanced diet rich in nutrients. Proper nutrition supports brain health and can influence your mood and emotional state.

Adequate Sleep:

Prioritize quality sleep as it directly impacts mental and emotional well-being. Lack of sleep can exacerbate stress and negatively affect your mood.

Mindfulness and Relaxation:

Incorporate mindfulness and relaxation techniques into your daily routine to reduce stress, increase self-awareness, and enhance emotional regulation.

Positive Relationships:

Healthy Boundaries:

Set and maintain healthy boundaries in your relationships to protect your mental and emotional well-being. Boundaries help ensure that your needs are respected.

Effective Communication:

Practice effective communication by expressing your thoughts and emotions openly and honestly. Encourage others to do the same, fostering understanding and empathy.

Conflict Resolution:

Develop conflict resolution skills to navigate disagreements constructively and prevent unresolved conflicts from negatively impacting your well-being.

Nurturing mental and emotional well-being is an ongoing process that requires self-awareness, self-compassion, and a commitment to self-care. By adopting these strategies and actively tending to your mental and emotional health, you empower yourself to lead a more fulfilling and balanced life, fostering a profound sense of well-being and happiness.

Nurturing Your Mental Health

Nurturing your mental health is a fundamental aspect of your wellness journey. Mental health plays a pivotal role in your overall well-being, affecting how you think, feel, and act. In this chapter, we shall explore strategies and practices to help you nurture and prioritize your mental health for a happier and more fulfilling life.

Self-Care for Mental Health:

Self-Compassion:

Treat yourself with the same kindness and understanding that you would offer to a friend. Practice self-compassion, especially during challenging times.

Stress Management:

Develop effective stress management techniques, such as deep breathing exercises, meditation, or yoga, to reduce the impact of stress on your mental health.

Regular Exercise:

Engage in regular physical activity, as it releases endorphins, which are natural mood lifters. Exercise also supports cognitive function and reduces stress.

Nutrition:

Maintain a balanced diet rich in nutrients, as proper nutrition is essential for brain health. Nutrient-dense foods can positively impact your mood and cognitive function.

Adequate Sleep:

Prioritize quality sleep, aiming for 7-9 hours per night. A well-rested mind is better equipped to cope with challenges and maintain emotional balance.

Emotional Regulation:

Mindfulness Practice:

Engage in mindfulness meditation to enhance your awareness of your thoughts and emotions. Mindfulness can help you manage your reactions to difficult emotions more effectively.

Emotion Expression:

Express your emotions in healthy ways, whether through journaling, talking to a trusted friend, or seeking professional counseling. Avoid bottling up your feelings, as it can lead to increased stress and mental strain.

Social Connections:

Maintain Relationships:

Cultivate and maintain strong social connections with friends and family. Positive relationships provide emotional support and a sense of belonging.

Effective Communication:

Practice effective communication in your relationships. Express your thoughts and feelings openly and listen empathetically to others. Healthy communication fosters understanding and reduces conflict.

Lifelong Learning and Growth:

Engage in New Experiences:

Continue to seek new experiences and challenges that stimulate your mind. Lifelong learning and personal growth contribute to a sense of purpose and well-being.

Set Goals:

Establish realistic and meaningful goals for yourself. Working toward objectives can enhance your sense of accomplishment and motivation.

Professional Guidance:

Seek Help When Needed:

If you're struggling with persistent mental health challenges, don't hesitate to seek the guidance of a mental health professional. Therapy or counseling can provide valuable tools and support.

Medication and Treatment:

If recommended by a healthcare professional, consider medication or other treatment options for mental health conditions. These interventions can play a crucial role in managing certain disorders.

Healthy Lifestyle Habits:

Limit Substance Use:

Use alcohol and other substances in moderation, if at all. Excessive substance use can negatively impact your mental health.

Mindfulness and Relaxation:

Incorporate mindfulness and relaxation techniques into your daily routine to reduce stress and promote emotional well-being.

Positive Self-Image:

Challenge Negative Thoughts:

Challenge and reframe negative self-talk. Replace self-criticism with self-compassion and positive affirmations.

Acceptance and Self-Love:

Embrace self-acceptance and self-love. Acknowledge that you are worthy of care and kindness, regardless of your perceived flaws or imperfections.

Community Involvement:

Volunteer and Give Back:

Engage in volunteer work or community activities. Giving back can foster a sense of purpose and connection to others.

Supportive Networks:

Join or create support networks and groups for shared interests or challenges. Connecting with like-minded individuals can provide a sense of belonging.

Nurturing your mental health is an ongoing and individualized journey. By prioritizing self-care, seeking support when needed, and adopting a holistic approach to well-being, you empower yourself to lead a mentally and emotionally healthy life. Remember that your mental health is an essential part of your overall wellness, and it deserves the same care and attention as your physical health.

Strategies for Stress Reduction

Stress reduction is a pivotal aspect of your wellness journey, promoting mental and physical well-being. In our fast-paced world, effective strategies to manage and alleviate stress are essential for a happier and healthier life. In this chapter, we shall explore a variety of stress reduction techniques to help you navigate life's challenges with grace and resilience.

Mindfulness and Relaxation Techniques:

Mindfulness Meditation:

Practice mindfulness meditation by focusing your attention on the present moment without judgment. Regular meditation cultivates awareness and reduces stress.

Deep Breathing Exercises:

Deep breathing exercises, such as diaphragmatic breathing,

can quickly induce relaxation. Inhale deeply through your nose, allowing your abdomen to rise, then exhale slowly through your mouth, releasing tension.

Progressive Muscle Relaxation:

Engage in progressive muscle relaxation by systematically tensing and then relaxing different muscle groups in your body. This technique promotes physical and mental relaxation.

Guided Imagery:

Guided imagery involves using your imagination to create a mental scene that promotes relaxation. Visualize a peaceful place or scenario, engaging all your senses to enhance the experience.

Body Scan Meditation:

Body scan meditation involves focusing your attention on each part of your body, starting from your toes and moving upward. It helps you become aware of physical sensations and release tension.

Lifestyle and Wellness Practices:

Regular Physical Activity:

Engaging in regular exercise is a potent stress reducer. It releases endorphins, improves mood, and helps your body manage stress more effectively.

Healthy Diet:

Maintain a balanced diet rich in nutrients. Proper nutrition supports brain health and can influence your mood and emotional state.

Adequate Sleep:

Prioritize quality sleep to recharge your body and mind. Lack of sleep can exacerbate stress and negatively affect your mood.

Mindful Rest Breaks:

Take short, mindful breaks during the day to recharge. Deep breathing, stretching, or a brief walk can help reduce stress and enhance your overall sense of well-being.

Positive Relationships:

Social Support:

Maintain strong social connections with friends and family. Sharing your thoughts and feelings with trusted individuals can provide emotional support and perspective.

Effective Communication:

Practice effective communication in your relationships. Express your thoughts and feelings openly and listen empathetically to others. Healthy communication fosters understanding and reduces conflict.

Time Management:

Prioritize and Organize:

Set priorities and organize your tasks. Effective time management can reduce stress related to work or daily responsibilities.

Set Realistic Goals:

Establish realistic and attainable goals for yourself. Unrealistic expectations can lead to unnecessary stress and frustration.

Professional Guidance:

Therapy and Counseling:

Consider seeking the guidance of a therapist or counselor, especially if you're dealing with chronic stress or specific stressors. They can provide coping strategies and support.

Mind-Body Therapies:

Mind-body therapies such as acupuncture, massage therapy, or biofeedback can complement stress management efforts and promote relaxation.

Limit Substance Use:

Moderation:

Use alcohol and other substances in moderation, if at all.

Excessive substance use can exacerbate stress and negatively impact your well-being.

Positive Self-Image:

Positive Self-Talk:

Challenge and reframe negative self-talk. Replace self-criticism with self-compassion and positive affirmations.

Acceptance and Self-Love:

Embrace self-acceptance and self-love. Acknowledge that you are worthy of care and kindness, regardless of your perceived flaws or imperfections.

Hobbies and Interests:

Engage in Enjoyable Activities:

Make time for hobbies and interests that bring you joy. Engaging in activities you love provides a natural source of stress relief.

Creativity:

Express your creativity through art, writing, music, or other creative pursuits. Creativity can be a therapeutic outlet for stress.

Stress reduction is a personal and ongoing journey. By incorporating these strategies into your daily life and customizing them to your specific needs, you empower yourself to effectively manage stress and cultivate a sense of balance and well-being. Remember that stress is a natural part of life, but with the right tools, you can navigate it with grace and resilience.

Cultivating Resilience and Emotional Intelligence

Cultivating resilience and emotional intelligence are essential skills on your journey toward a happier and healthier life. These skills empower you to navigate life's challenges with grace, adaptability, and emotional well-being. In this chapter, we shall explore the significance of resilience and emotional intelligence and provide strategies to nurture and enhance them.

Understanding Resilience:

Resilience is the ability to bounce back from adversity, adapt to change, and effectively cope with stress and challenges. It's not about avoiding difficult situations but rather about developing the inner strength to face them.

Strategies for Cultivating Resilience:

Positive Self-Image:

Cultivate a positive self-image by acknowledging your strengths and accomplishments. Self-confidence and self-esteem are foundations of resilience.

Optimism:

Foster an optimistic outlook by focusing on solutions rather than problems. Maintain a hopeful perspective, even in the face of adversity.

Adaptability:

Embrace change as a natural part of life. Cultivate adaptability by learning to adjust to new circumstances and challenges.

Problem-Solving Skills:

Develop problem-solving skills to approach difficulties with a solution-oriented mindset. Break challenges into manageable steps and seek creative solutions.

Social Support:

Build and maintain strong social connections. Support from friends and family provides emotional strength during tough times.

Emotional Regulation:

Practice emotional regulation by acknowledging and managing your emotions effectively. This enables you to respond to stressors with composure.

Understanding Emotional Intelligence:

Emotional intelligence (EI) refers to the ability to recognize, understand, manage, and effectively use your emotions and those of others. It plays a vital role in building positive relationships, making sound decisions, and fostering well-being.

Strategies for Enhancing Emotional Intelligence:

Self-Awareness:

Develop self-awareness by regularly reflecting on your thoughts, feelings, and behaviors. Understand how your emotions influence your actions.

Self-Regulation:

Practice self-regulation by managing your emotional reactions. Avoid impulsive decisions driven by strong emotions, and cultivate emotional balance.

Empathy:

Enhance empathy by actively listening to others and trying to understand their perspectives and emotions. Empathy fosters understanding and compassion.

Effective Communication:

Practice effective communication by expressing your thoughts and emotions openly and empathetically. This encourages open dialogue and reduces misunderstandings.

Conflict Resolution:

Develop conflict resolution skills to navigate disagreements constructively. Focus on finding mutually beneficial solutions rather than escalating conflicts.

Social Skills:

Improve your social skills by building positive relationships and effective interpersonal communication. Social skills are crucial for maintaining healthy connections.

Cultivating Resilience and Emotional Intelligence in Daily Life:

Mindfulness and Self-Reflection:

Engage in mindfulness practices to increase self-awareness and emotional regulation. Regular self-reflection can help you identify areas for improvement.

Positive Relationships:

Foster positive relationships by practicing empathy and effective communication. Healthy connections provide emotional support and opportunities for growth.

Challenging Situations:

View challenging situations as opportunities to cultivate resilience and emotional intelligence. Embrace difficulties as chances for personal growth.

Seeking Professional Help:

If you're facing particularly challenging emotional issues or need guidance on enhancing emotional intelligence, consider consulting a mental health professional or therapist.

Cultivating resilience and emotional intelligence is a lifelong journey. By integrating these skills into your daily life and continuously refining them, you empower yourself to face life's uncertainties with poise and empathy. These skills not only enhance your own well-being but also contribute to more harmonious relationships and a deeper understanding of the human experience.

6

Chapter 6

Social Connections and Support

Social connections and support are invaluable components of your wellness journey, contributing significantly to your emotional well-being and overall quality of life. In this chapter, we shall explore the importance of social connections, the benefits of social support, and strategies to cultivate and nurture meaningful relationships.

Understanding Social Connections:

Social Bonds:

Social connections encompass relationships with friends, family, colleagues, and community members. These bonds provide a sense of belonging and connection to the world around you.

Emotional Well-Being:

Positive social interactions are closely linked to emotional well-being. Meaningful relationships offer emotional support, reduce stress, and promote happiness.

Benefits of Social Support:

Emotional Support:

Friends and family provide emotional support during challenging times, offering a listening ear, empathy, and comfort.

Stress Reduction:

Strong social connections can help reduce the physiological and psychological effects of stress. Sharing your burdens with others can lighten the load.

Mental Health:

Maintaining social connections is associated with improved mental health. Loneliness and social isolation, on the other hand, are risk factors for mental health issues.

Physical Health:

Social support is linked to better physical health outcomes. It can boost immunity, lower blood pressure, and promote longevity.

Sense of Belonging:

Social connections provide a sense of belonging and purpose, reinforcing your identity as part of a larger community.

Cultivating and Nurturing Social Connections:

Quality Over Quantity:

Focus on the quality of your relationships rather than the quantity. Meaningful connections provide more significant benefits than a large social network.

Active Listening:

Practice active listening when engaging with others. Show genuine interest in their thoughts and feelings, and avoid interrupting or judging.

Reciprocity:

Nurture give-and-take relationships. Offer support to others when they need it, and don't hesitate to seek support when you require it.

Shared Interests:

Connect with others who share your interests and passions. Common activities and hobbies provide a natural foundation for forming connections.

Community Involvement:

Engage in community activities, clubs, or volunteer work to meet like-minded individuals and build a sense of belonging.

Technology and Social Media:

Use technology and social media mindfully to maintain and strengthen relationships. Virtual connections can be valuable, but they should complement, not replace, in-person interactions.

Strengthening Existing Relationships:

Communication:

Maintain open and honest communication with your loved ones. Address conflicts and misunderstandings proactively to prevent them from escalating.

Quality Time:

Spend quality time with friends and family, engaging in activities that foster connection and bonding.

Celebrate Milestones:

Acknowledge and celebrate important milestones and achievements of your loved ones. Showing support during their successes strengthens your relationships.

Seeking Professional Help:

Therapy or Counseling:

If you're facing challenges in your relationships or struggling with social isolation, consider seeking the guidance of a therapist or counselor. They can provide strategies and support.

Support Groups:

Join support groups or therapy groups that address specific issues or challenges you may be facing. These groups offer a safe space for sharing experiences and connecting with others.

Balancing Independence and Connection:

Self-Care:

Prioritize self-care to maintain your emotional well-being. It's important to strike a balance between maintaining social connections and taking time for yourself.

Boundaries:

Set healthy boundaries in your relationships to ensure your own well-being is respected. Boundaries help prevent burnout and maintain harmony.

Maintaining Long-Distance Relationships:

Regular Communication:

Stay in touch with loved ones who are far away through regular communication. Video calls, emails, and handwritten letters can bridge the gap.

Scheduled Visits:

Plan visits and reunions to maintain a sense of closeness and connection with long-distance friends and family.

Social connections and support are integral to your wellness journey. By recognizing the importance of these connections, nurturing existing relationships, and actively seeking opportunities to connect with others, you enhance your emotional well-being and create a support network that can uplift you during life's challenges and celebrate your successes.

The Importance of Social Wellness

Social wellness is a vital dimension of your overall well-being, playing a significant role in your happiness and quality of life. In this chapter, we shall delve into the importance of social wellness, its impact on your mental and physical health, and strategies to cultivate and maintain a socially fulfilling life.

Understanding Social Wellness:

Social wellness encompasses the quality and richness of your social connections and relationships. It involves maintaining healthy and positive interactions with others, fostering a sense of belonging, and experiencing a supportive and fulfilling social life.

The Impact of Social Wellness:

Emotional Well-Being:

Positive social interactions contribute to emotional well-being by providing emotional support, reducing stress, and promoting feelings of happiness and contentment.

Mental Health:

Strong social connections are closely linked to improved mental health. Loneliness and social isolation, on the other hand, can increase the risk of mental health issues such as depression and anxiety.

Physical Health:

Social wellness has a profound impact on physical health. Studies show that individuals with strong social support networks tend to have better immune function, lower blood pressure, and reduced risk of chronic diseases.

Stress Reduction:

Social support acts as a buffer against the negative effects of stress. Sharing your concerns and challenges with trusted friends and family members can alleviate stress and promote resilience.

Sense of Belonging:

A robust social network fosters a sense of belonging and connection to a larger community. Feeling part of a supportive group enhances self-esteem and provides a sense of purpose.

Longevity:

Research suggests that individuals with active social lives tend to live longer, healthier lives. Socially engaged people are more likely to adopt healthy behaviors and seek medical attention when needed.

Strategies for Cultivating Social Wellness:

Nurture Existing Relationships:

Invest time and effort in maintaining and strengthening your current relationships with friends, family, and colleagues. Quality connections require care and attention.

Active Listening:

Practice active listening when engaging with others. Show genuine interest in their thoughts and feelings, and avoid interrupting or judging.

Reciprocity:

Cultivate give-and-take relationships. Offer support to others when they need it, and don't hesitate to seek support when you require it.

Shared Interests:

Connect with others who share your interests and passions. Common activities and hobbies provide a natural foundation for forming connections.

Community Involvement:

Engage in community activities, clubs, or volunteer work to meet like-minded individuals and build a sense of belonging.

Technology and Social Media:

Use technology and social media mindfully to maintain and strengthen relationships. Virtual connections can be valuable, but they should complement, not replace, in-person interactions.

Strengthening Existing Relationships:

Maintain open and honest communication with your loved ones. Address conflicts and misunderstandings proactively to prevent them from escalating.

Celebrate Milestones:

Acknowledge and celebrate important milestones and achievements of your loved ones. Showing support during their successes strengthens your relationships.

Seeking Professional Help:

Therapy or Counseling:

If you're facing challenges in your relationships or struggling with social isolation, consider seeking the guidance of a therapist or counselor. They can provide strategies and support.

Support Groups:

Join support groups or therapy groups that address specific issues or challenges you may be facing. These groups offer a safe space for sharing experiences and connecting with others.

Balancing Independence and Connection:

Self-Care:

Prioritize self-care to maintain your emotional well-being. It's important to strike a balance between maintaining social connections and taking time for yourself.

Boundaries:

Set healthy boundaries in your relationships to ensure your own well-being is respected. Boundaries help prevent burnout and maintain harmony.

Social wellness is an integral part of your wellness journey. By recognizing its significance, nurturing existing relationships, and actively seeking opportunities to connect with others, you enhance your emotional well-being and create a support network that can uplift you during life's challenges and celebrate your successes.

Building Healthy Relationships

Building and maintaining healthy relationships is a cornerstone of your wellness journey. Healthy relationships are essential for emotional well-being, happiness, and personal growth. In this chapter, we shall explore the principles of healthy relationships and provide strategies to cultivate and sustain them.

Principles of Healthy Relationships:

Communication:

Open and honest communication is the foundation of healthy relationships. Effective communication involves active listening, expressing thoughts and feelings respectfully, and addressing conflicts constructively.

Respect:

Mutual respect is key. Treat each other with kindness and consideration, valuing each person's opinions, boundaries, and individuality.

Trust:

Trust forms the bedrock of any healthy relationship. Be reliable and trustworthy, and trust your partner or friend in return. Trust is earned and maintained over time.

Support:

Healthy relationships provide emotional support during challenging times and celebrate each other's successes. Be there for your loved ones when they need you.

Equality:

Healthy relationships are built on equality. No one should dominate or control the other. Each person's opinions and feelings should be equally valued.

Independence and Togetherness:

Balance the need for independence with the desire for togetherness. Healthy relationships allow each person to maintain their individuality while sharing a meaningful connection.

Boundaries:

Set and respect healthy boundaries in your relationships. Boundaries define what is acceptable and what isn't, promoting mutual understanding and respect.

Strategies for Building Healthy Relationships:

Effective Communication:

Practice active listening, empathy, and assertiveness in your communication. Ensure that both you and your partner or friend feel heard and understood.

Conflict Resolution:

Develop conflict resolution skills. Address disagreements calmly, focusing on finding solutions rather than placing blame.

Quality Time:

Spend quality time together to nurture your connection. Engage in activities you both enjoy and create shared memories.

Appreciation and Gratitude:

Express appreciation and gratitude for your loved ones regularly. Small gestures of kindness and acknowledgment can strengthen bonds.

Support Each Other's Goals:

Encourage and support each other's personal and professional goals. Celebrate each other's achievements and provide encouragement during challenges.

Share Responsibilities:

Share responsibilities in your relationships, whether in a romantic partnership or friendship. Fair distribution of tasks fosters a sense of partnership and teamwork.

Empathy and Understanding:

Cultivate empathy and understanding. Try to see things from

the other person's perspective, even if you don't agree. This promotes compassion and connection.

Apologize and Forgive:

Be willing to apologize when you make mistakes and forgive others when they do. Holding onto grudges can erode the foundation of a healthy relationship.

Seeking Professional Help:

Couples or Family Therapy:

If you're facing persistent issues in your relationships, consider couples or family therapy. A trained therapist can help you navigate challenges and improve communication.

Friendship Counseling:

For complex friendship dynamics, friendship counseling or support groups can provide valuable insights and strategies for healthier friendships.

Healthy Relationships with Yourself:

Self-Care:

Prioritize self-care and self-compassion. Building a healthy relationship with yourself is the foundation for healthy relationships with others.

Set Boundaries:

Set and enforce healthy boundaries in all your relationships, including the one with yourself. Self-respect is essential.

Positive Self-Talk:

Challenge negative self-talk and cultivate self-love and self-acceptance. A positive self-relationship enhances your ability to have positive relationships with others.

Seek Personal Growth:

Engage in personal growth and self-improvement. A fulfilling relationship with yourself involves continuous self-discovery and development.

Building and maintaining healthy relationships is an ongoing process that requires effort and commitment. By applying these principles and strategies, you empower yourself to create and sustain meaningful connections that contribute to your overall well-being and happiness.

Seeking Support and Community

Seeking support and community is a valuable aspect of your wellness journey. It allows you to connect with others who share your experiences, challenges, and goals, providing a sense of belonging and a source of encouragement. In this chapter, we shall explore the importance of seeking support and community, the benefits it offers, and strategies to find and engage with supportive networks.

Understanding the Importance of Support and Community:

Emotional Well-Being:

Seeking support and community can significantly impact your emotional well-being. It offers a space to share your thoughts and feelings, reducing feelings of isolation and loneliness.

Validation and Understanding:

Connecting with others who have similar experiences can provide validation and understanding. It helps you realize that you're not alone in facing your challenges.

Motivation and Encouragement:

Supportive networks and communities can motivate and encourage you to pursue your goals and maintain a positive outlook, even during challenging times.

Personal Growth:

Engaging with like-minded individuals can promote personal growth by exposing you to new perspectives and opportunities for learning and development.

Problem-Solving:

Supportive networks often offer valuable insights and advice for problem-solving. Collaborating with others can lead to creative solutions to common challenges.

Strategies for Seeking Support and Community:

Identify Your Needs:

Reflect on your needs and goals. Consider the areas of your life where support and community can be most beneficial.

Join Interest-Based Groups:

Seek out clubs, organizations, or online communities that align with your interests and passions. Sharing common hobbies is an excellent way to connect with like-minded individuals.

Local or Virtual Support Groups:

Explore local or virtual support groups that address specific issues or challenges you may be facing. These groups provide a safe space for sharing experiences and connecting with others.

Social Media and Online Forums:

Utilize social media and online forums to find and engage with communities that resonate with your interests or needs. Many platforms host niche groups and forums for various topics.

Attend Workshops and Events:

Attend workshops, seminars, or events related to your interests or goals. These gatherings offer opportunities to connect with others who share your passions.

Volunteer:

Consider volunteering for causes or organizations that align with your values. Volunteering not only provides a sense of purpose but also connects you with a community of like-hearted individuals.

Professional Networks:

Join professional networks and associations related to your field of work or study. These networks can facilitate career development and offer valuable support.

Effective Engagement with Support and Community:

Active Participation:

Actively participate in your chosen communities or support groups. Engage in discussions, share your experiences, and offer support to others.

Respect and Empathy:

Approach interactions with respect and empathy. Understand that everyone has their unique experiences and challenges.

Reciprocity:

Foster give-and-take relationships within your support networks. Be willing to offer assistance and support when needed, and don't hesitate to seek help when you require it.

Boundaries:

Set and respect boundaries within your communities. Boundaries ensure that your well-being is protected and that interactions remain respectful.

Professional Guidance:

Therapy or Counseling:

If you're dealing with specific issues or seeking personal growth, consider individual therapy or counseling. A trained professional can provide guidance and support tailored to your needs.

Life Coaching:

Life coaching can be a valuable resource for setting and achieving personal or professional goals. Coaches provide accountability and strategies for success.

Seeking support and community is a proactive step toward enhancing your well-being and personal growth. By identifying your needs, actively engaging with supportive networks, and approaching interactions with respect and empathy, you empower yourself to find connections that enrich your life and contribute to your overall happiness and fulfillment.

7

Chapter 7

Balancing Work and Life

Balancing work and life is essential for your overall well-being and long-term happiness. Striking this equilibrium allows you to excel in your professional pursuits while maintaining a fulfilling personal life. In this chapter, we shall explore the significance of work-life balance, its impact on your health and relationships, and strategies to achieve and maintain it.

Understanding Work-Life Balance:

Work-life balance refers to the equilibrium between your professional responsibilities and personal life outside of work. Achieving this balance is crucial for your physical and mental health, as well as your relationships.

The Impact of Work-Life Balance:

Mental Health:

Maintaining work-life balance is essential for your mental health. An imbalance, with excessive work demands, can lead to stress, burnout, and a decline in psychological well-being.

Physical Health:

Work-life balance has a direct impact on your physical health. Prolonged periods of overwork can lead to exhaustion, sleep problems, and increased risk of health issues.

Relationships:

A balanced life allows you to nurture and sustain meaningful relationships with family and friends. Neglecting personal connections due to work commitments can strain relationships.

Productivity and Creativity:

Striking a balance can enhance your productivity and creativity at work. Rest and personal time are essential for rejuvenation and fresh perspectives.

Strategies for Achieving Work-Life Balance:

Prioritize Self-Care:

Make self-care a non-negotiable part of your routine. Prioritize activities that rejuvenate your mind and body, such as exercise, meditation, or hobbies.

Set Boundaries:

Set clear boundaries between work and personal life. Establish specific work hours and avoid bringing work-related tasks or stress home.

Time Management:

Efficient time management is crucial. Prioritize tasks, delegate when possible, and avoid overcommitting yourself.

Use Technology Mindfully:

Be mindful of your use of technology, especially outside of work hours. Consider setting boundaries for checking emails or messages.

Scheduling Personal Time:

Schedule personal time in your calendar, just as you would for work meetings. This ensures that you allocate time for self-care and personal pursuits.

Delegate and Seek Help:

Don't hesitate to delegate tasks or seek help when needed, whether at work or home. Sharing responsibilities lightens your load.

Learn to Say No:

Learn to say no to additional work or commitments that can compromise your work-life balance. It's okay to decline when it's not feasible.

Vacation and Downtime:

Take regular vacations and downtime. Disconnect from work during these periods to recharge fully.

Flexible Work Arrangements:

Explore flexible work arrangements if your job allows, such as remote work or adjusted hours. Discuss these options with your employer.

Evaluate Your Priorities:

Reflect on your values and priorities. Ensure that your work aligns with your long-term goals and values.

Maintaining Work-Life Balance:

Regular Assessment:

Regularly assess your work-life balance. If you notice an imbalance, take steps to adjust and restore equilibrium.

Open Communication:

Communicate with your employer, colleagues, and loved ones about your work-life balance goals and needs. Open communication fosters understanding and support.

Adaptability:

Be adaptable and willing to adjust your approach to work-life balance as your circumstances change. Life is dynamic, and your balance may need occasional adjustments.

Seek Professional Guidance:

If you're struggling to achieve work-life balance due to specific challenges, consider consulting a coach or therapist who specializes in work-life balance issues.

Achieving and maintaining work-life balance is a continuous process that requires conscious effort and self-awareness. By implementing these strategies and prioritizing self-care and personal time, you empower yourself to lead a more fulfilling life that encompasses both professional success and personal happiness.

Achieving Work-Life Balance

Achieving work-life balance is a fundamental aspect of your wellness journey, allowing you to lead a fulfilling life that encompasses both professional success and personal well-being. In this chapter, we shall delve into practical strategies and principles to help you achieve and maintain a harmonious work-life balance.

Understanding Work-Life Balance:

Work-life balance involves effectively managing your professional responsibilities and personal life, ensuring that neither one overshadows the other. Striking this equilibrium is essential for your physical and mental health, as well as your overall happiness.

Principles for Achieving Work-Life Balance:

Prioritization:

Identify your top priorities in both your professional and personal life. This clarity helps you allocate time and energy effectively.

Boundaries:

Set clear boundaries between work and personal life. Define specific work hours, and avoid letting work encroach into your personal time.

Time Management:

Practice efficient time management. Prioritize tasks, delegate when possible, and avoid overcommitting yourself.

Self-Care:

Prioritize self-care as a non-negotiable part of your routine. Engage in activities that rejuvenate your mind and body, such as exercise, meditation, or hobbies.

Technology Mindfulness:

Be mindful of your use of technology, especially outside of work hours. Set boundaries for checking emails and messages.

Delegation:

Don't hesitate to delegate tasks or seek help when needed, both at work and home. Sharing responsibilities lightens your load.

Effective Communication:

Communicate openly with your employer, colleagues, and loved ones about your work-life balance goals and needs. Effective communication fosters understanding and support.

Learning to Say No:

Learn to say no to additional work or commitments that can compromise your work-life balance. It's okay to decline when it's not feasible.

Strategies for Achieving and Maintaining Work-Life Balance:

Scheduled Personal Time:

Schedule personal time in your calendar, treating it with the same importance as work commitments. This ensures that you allocate time for self-care and personal pursuits.

Vacation and Downtime:

Take regular vacations and downtime. Disconnect from work

during these periods to fully recharge.

Flexible Work Arrangements:

Explore flexible work arrangements if your job allows, such as remote work or adjusted hours. Discuss these options with your employer.

Evaluation and Adjustment:

Regularly assess your work-life balance. If you notice an imbalance, take proactive steps to adjust and restore equilibrium.

Adaptability:

Be adaptable and willing to adjust your approach to work-life balance as your circumstances change. Life is dynamic, and your balance may need occasional adjustments.

Seek Professional Guidance:

If you're struggling to achieve work-life balance due to specific challenges or stressors, consider consulting a coach or therapist who specializes in work-life balance issues.

Balancing Work and Personal Goals:

Reflect on Your Values:

Reflect on your values and priorities in both your professional and personal life. Ensure that your work aligns with your long-term goals and values.

Plan for Personal Growth:

Invest in personal growth and self-improvement. Balancing work and personal life becomes more manageable when you're continually evolving and growing.

Achieving and maintaining work-life balance is an ongoing process that requires dedication and self-awareness. By implementing these principles and strategies, you empower yourself to lead a more fulfilling life that encompasses both professional success and personal happiness.

Time Management for Wellness

Effective time management is a cornerstone of your wellness journey. It empowers you to make the most of your time, reduce stress, and create a balance between work, personal life, and self-care. In this chapter, we shall explore the importance of time management for wellness, principles to enhance it, and strategies to make the most of your time.

Understanding the Importance of Time Management for Wellness:

Time is a finite resource, and how you manage it significantly impacts your well-being. Effective time management can:

Reduce Stress:

Organizing your time reduces the stress associated with missed deadlines and overwhelming tasks.

Enhance Productivity:

Prioritizing tasks and managing your time efficiently leads to increased productivity, freeing up time for self-care and personal pursuits.

Create Balance:

Balancing work, personal life, and self-care allows you to lead a more fulfilling and balanced life.

Boost Well-Being:

Time management contributes to your overall well-being by allowing you to allocate time to activities that promote physical, mental, and emotional health.

Principles for Effective Time Management:

Prioritization:

Identify your top priorities and allocate time accordingly. Focus on what truly matters.

Goal Setting:

Set clear and achievable goals. Goals provide direction and motivation for your tasks.

Task Organization:

Organize tasks by importance and urgency. Use tools like to-do lists or digital apps to keep track of your responsibilities.

Time Blocking:

Allocate specific time blocks for different tasks or activities. This helps you stay focused and prevents multitasking.

Minimize Distractions:

Identify common distractions and take steps to minimize them during work or focused tasks.

Learn to Say No:

Practice saying no to additional commitments or tasks that may derail your priorities.

Self-Care Allocation:

Prioritize self-care by scheduling time for exercise, relaxation, hobbies, and spending time with loved ones.

Strategies for Effective Time Management:

Daily Planning:

Begin each day with a plan. Outline your tasks and goals for the day, including work-related responsibilities and personal pursuits.

Weekly and Monthly Planning:

Extend your planning to a weekly and monthly level. Set objectives for the week and month to ensure you're progressing toward your long-term goals.

Time Audit:

Conduct a time audit to assess how you're currently spending your time. Identify areas where you can reallocate time for wellness activities.

Time Tracking Apps:

Use time tracking apps or tools to monitor your activities and identify time-wasting habits.

Delegate and Outsource:

Delegate tasks that others can handle, both in your personal and professional life. Consider outsourcing tasks that don't require your direct involvement.

Batching:

Group similar tasks together and tackle them in dedicated time blocks. Batching increases efficiency and minimizes context switching.

Limit Meetings and Distractions:

Set specific times for meetings and limit their duration. Minimize interruptions by turning off non-essential notifications.

Set Deadlines:

Establish self-imposed deadlines for tasks to create a sense of urgency and focus.

Regular Breaks:

Incorporate regular breaks into your work routine to recharge and maintain productivity.

Review and Adjust:

Periodically review your time management strategies and make adjustments as needed to ensure they align with your goals and priorities.

Balancing Work, Personal Life, and Self-Care:

Block Personal Time:

Schedule personal time for self-care, family, and leisure activities, treating them with the same importance as work commitments.

Unplug and Disconnect:

Set boundaries for technology use to disconnect from work and allow time for personal and self-care activities.

Self-Care Rituals:

Establish self-care rituals that promote wellness, such as daily meditation, exercise routines, or relaxation practices.

Quality Time:

Focus on the quality of your interactions with loved ones during personal time, rather than quantity.

Delegate and Share Responsibilities:

Share responsibilities with family members or housemates to ensure a fair distribution of tasks.

Effective time management is a learned skill that requires practice and adjustment. By embracing these principles and implementing strategies that align with your goals, you'll enhance your ability to manage your time effectively, reduce stress, and prioritize wellness in your daily life.

Avoiding Burnout

Avoiding burnout is a crucial aspect of your wellness journey, ensuring that you can sustain high levels of productivity and well-being over the long term. Burnout can have detrimental effects on your physical and mental health, as well as your overall satisfaction with life. In this chapter, we shall explore the importance of avoiding burnout, the signs to watch for, and strategies to prevent and recover from it.

Understanding the Importance of Avoiding Burnout:

Burnout is a state of physical, emotional, and mental exhaustion resulting from prolonged exposure to excessive stress and overwork. It can lead to a range of negative consequences, including:

Physical Health Issues:

Burnout is associated with a higher risk of various health problems, such as cardiovascular disease, weakened immune system, and chronic fatigue.

Mental Health Challenges:

Prolonged burnout can lead to anxiety, depression, and other mental health disorders.

Decreased Job Performance:

Burnout negatively impacts your job performance, leading to decreased productivity, increased errors, and a lack of motivation.

Strained Relationships:

Burnout can spill over into your personal life, straining relationships with family and friends due to increased irritability and reduced engagement.

Signs of Burnout:

Recognizing the signs of burnout is crucial for taking proactive steps to prevent or address it. Common signs of burnout include:

Chronic Fatigue:

Feeling constantly tired, both physically and mentally, despite getting adequate rest.

Reduced Concentration:

Difficulty focusing on tasks and reduced attention span.

Cynicism and Detachment:

Developing a negative and cynical attitude towards work or life in general.

Decreased Productivity:

A noticeable decline in productivity and effectiveness in your tasks.

Increased Irritability:

Becoming easily frustrated or irritable, both at work and in personal relationships.

Physical Symptoms:

Experiencing physical symptoms like headaches, gastrointestinal issues, or sleep disturbances.

Loss of Interest:

A loss of interest in activities or tasks that once brought enjoyment.

Strategies for Avoiding Burnout:

Self-Care:

Prioritize self-care by allocating time for relaxation, exercise, hobbies, and activities that rejuvenate your mind and body.

Set Boundaries:

Set clear boundaries between work and personal life. Define specific work hours and avoid bringing work-related tasks or stress home.

Time Management:

Practice efficient time management to prevent overwhelming workloads. Prioritize tasks, delegate when possible, and avoid overcommitting yourself.

Seek Support:

Seek support from friends, family, or a therapist if you're feeling overwhelmed. Talking about your feelings can provide relief and perspective.

Regular Breaks:

Incorporate regular breaks into your work routine to recharge and prevent burnout.

Limit Technology Use:

Set boundaries for technology use to disconnect from work during personal and self-care time.

Delegate and Share Responsibilities:

Share responsibilities with family members or housemates to ensure a fair distribution of tasks.

Goal Setting:

Set clear and achievable goals, both at work and in your personal life, to provide direction and motivation.

Evaluate Priorities:

Reflect on your values and priorities, ensuring that your commitments align with your long-term goals and well-being.

Practice Mindfulness:

Incorporate mindfulness and relaxation practices into your daily routine to manage stress and stay grounded.

Recovering from Burnout:

If you suspect you're already experiencing burnout, consider the following steps for recovery:

Seek Professional Help:

Consult a therapist or counselor who specializes in burnout and stress management. Professional guidance can be invaluable in recovery.

Take a Break:

If possible, take a temporary break from work to focus on your recovery. Rest and self-care are essential.

Reflect and Reevaluate:

Reflect on the factors that led to burnout and reevaluate your priorities and work-life balance.

Gradual Return to Work:

When you're ready, ease back into work gradually, with a focus on maintaining a healthy work-life balance.

Continuous Self-Care:

Commit to ongoing self-care practices to prevent future burnout.

Avoiding burnout is essential for your overall well-being and long-term success in both your professional and personal life. By recognizing the signs, implementing preventive strategies, and seeking support when needed, you empower yourself to maintain balance and wellness on your journey.

8

Chapter 8

Sustainable Health Habits

Sustainable health habits are the foundation of a long and ful-filling wellness journey. These habits not only promote physical well-being but also contribute to mental and emotional balance. In this chapter, we shall explore the significance of sustainable health habits, principles to develop them, and strategies to integrate them into your daily life.

Understanding the Importance of Sustainable Health Habits:

Sustainable health habits are practices that you can maintain consistently over time, leading to lasting well-being and vitality. These habits are vital because:

Long-Term Well-Being:

Sustainable health habits are not quick fixes; they are the building blocks of long-term well-being and resilience.

Holistic Wellness:

These habits encompass physical, mental, and emotional health, promoting a balanced and holistic approach to wellness.

Prevention:

They help prevent chronic diseases and health issues, reducing the risk of illness and improving your quality of life.

Stress Reduction:

Sustainable health habits provide tools to manage stress and enhance your ability to cope with life's challenges.

Principles for Developing Sustainable Health Habits:

Start Small:

Begin with small, manageable changes in your daily routine. Gradual adjustments are more likely to become lasting habits.

Consistency:

Consistency is key to developing sustainable habits. Commit to your chosen practices regularly.

Mindfulness:

Practice mindfulness in your daily life. Be aware of your choices and their impact on your well-being.

Personalization:

Tailor your health habits to your unique needs and preferences. What works for one person may not work for another.

Self-Compassion:

Be kind to yourself on your wellness journey. Avoid self-criticism and practice self-compassion.

Strategies for Integrating Sustainable Health Habits:

Healthy Eating:

Incorporate a balanced and nutritious diet into your daily life. Focus on whole foods, fruits, vegetables, lean proteins, and whole grains.

Regular Exercise:

Engage in regular physical activity that you enjoy. Find activities that fit your lifestyle and make exercise a fun part of your routine.

Adequate Sleep:

Prioritize quality sleep by establishing a consistent sleep schedule and creating a sleep-friendly environment.

Stress Management:

Learn and practice stress management techniques such as meditation, deep breathing, or yoga to build resilience.

Mindful Eating:

Practice mindful eating by paying attention to what you eat and savoring each bite. Avoid emotional eating or overindulgence.

Hydration:

Stay hydrated throughout the day by drinking plenty of water. Limit sugary beverages and excessive caffeine.

Regular Check-Ups:

Schedule regular check-ups with healthcare professionals to monitor your health and catch potential issues early.

Mental Health Care:

Prioritize your mental health by seeking therapy or counseling when needed. Develop healthy coping strategies for stress and emotions.

Social Connections:

Nurture social connections and maintain supportive relationships with friends and loved ones.

Hobbies and Recreation:

Make time for hobbies and recreational activities that bring joy and relaxation into your life.

Implementing Sustainable Health Habits:

Gradual Integration:

Introduce one new habit at a time. Once it becomes ingrained, add another one.

Accountability:

Find an accountability partner or support system to help you stay on track with your health habits.

Track Your Progress:

Keep a journal or use apps to track your progress and celebrate your successes.

Adaptability:

Be adaptable and willing to adjust your habits as your life circumstances change.

Seek Professional Guidance:

Consult healthcare professionals, nutritionists, or fitness trainers for personalized guidance on your health journey.

Developing sustainable health habits is a lifelong process that requires dedication and self-compassion. By applying these principles and strategies, you empower yourself to create a solid foundation for lasting well-being and vitality.

Habit Formation and Maintenance

Habit formation and maintenance are pivotal aspects of your wellness journey. These habits serve as the building blocks for long-term well-being and vitality. In this chapter, we shall explore the science behind habit formation, principles to develop and maintain habits effectively, and strategies to integrate them seamlessly into your daily life.

Understanding the Science of Habit Formation:

Habits are automatic behaviors that occur without conscious thought. They are formed through a process called the habit loop, which consists of three stages:

Cue: This is the trigger or stimulus that initiates the habit. It can be a specific time, place, emotion, or situation.

Routine: The routine is the behavior or action that follows the cue. It's the actual habit you're trying to establish.

Reward: The reward is the positive outcome or satisfaction you gain from completing the routine. It reinforces the habit loop.

Principles for Effective Habit Formation:

Start Small:

Begin with small, manageable changes in your daily routine. This makes it easier to establish new habits.

Consistency:

Consistency is crucial for habit formation. Commit to practicing your chosen habits regularly.

Set Clear Goals:

Define clear and specific goals for your habits. Knowing what you're aiming for helps you stay motivated.

Mindfulness:

Be mindful of your habits as you practice them. Pay attention to the cue, routine, and reward to better understand and modify your habits.

Track Your Progress:

Keep a record of your habit-building journey. Tracking your progress helps you stay accountable and motivated.

Strategies for Habit Formation and Maintenance:

Identify Your Cues:

Recognize the cues or triggers that lead to your desired habits. Understanding your triggers helps you anticipate and respond to them.

Create a Routine:

Develop a specific routine or action that you'll perform consistently in response to the cue.

Choose Meaningful Rewards:

Select rewards that are meaningful and motivating to you. Positive reinforcement strengthens the habit loop.

Stack Habits:

Pair your new habit with an existing one. This helps you remember to practice it and makes it easier to integrate into your routine.

Practice Gradual Progress:

Incrementally increase the difficulty or intensity of your habit as you become more comfortable with it.

Accountability:

Share your goals and progress with a friend or family member who can hold you accountable.

Visual Cues:

Use visual cues, such as sticky notes or reminders on your phone, to prompt habit execution.

Celebrate Milestones:

Celebrate your achievements and milestones along your habit-building journey. Acknowledging your progress reinforces positive behavior.

Overcoming Challenges in Habit Formation:

Habit Relapse:

If you lapse or miss a day, don't be discouraged. It's normal to experience setbacks. Revisit your motivation and continue.

Resistance to Change:

Embrace discomfort and resistance as part of the habit-building process. Change often feels challenging initially.

Lack of Motivation:

Reconnect with your underlying motivations and goals to reignite your enthusiasm for building and maintaining habits.

External Support:

Seek support from friends, family, or a coach to help you overcome challenges and stay on track.

Adaptability:

Be flexible and willing to adjust your habits as needed. Life circumstances may require adaptation.

Habit formation and maintenance are ongoing processes that require patience and perseverance. By applying these principles and strategies, you empower yourself to establish and sustain healthy habits that contribute to your overall well-being and vitality.

Overcoming Common Obstacles

Overcoming common obstacles is an integral part of your wellness journey. Challenges are inevitable, but they offer opportunities for growth and resilience. In this chapter, we shall explore common obstacles to wellness, strategies to overcome them, and the importance of perseverance in the face of adversity.

Understanding Common Obstacles to Wellness:

Time Constraints:

Busy schedules and work commitments can make it challenging to allocate time for self-care and wellness practices.

Procrastination:

Putting off healthy habits or tasks can hinder progress and lead to frustration.

Lack of Motivation:

Maintaining motivation for wellness activities can be difficult, especially when faced with setbacks or slow progress.

Stress and Overwhelm:

High levels of stress and overwhelm can make it challenging to focus on self-care and healthy habits.

Lack of Support:

Insufficient support from family, friends, or colleagues can hinder your wellness efforts.

Self-Doubt:

Negative self-talk and self-doubt can undermine your confidence and motivation.

Strategies for Overcoming Common Obstacles:

Time Management:

Prioritize time management to create space for wellness activities. Schedule self-care as you would any other appointment.

Goal Setting:

Set clear and achievable wellness goals. Having a purpose helps maintain motivation.

Break Tasks Into Smaller Steps:

When faced with a daunting task, break it into smaller, manageable steps to reduce overwhelm.

Accountability:

Share your wellness goals with a friend, family member, or coach who can provide support and accountability.

Mindfulness and Resilience:

Practice mindfulness and resilience-building techniques to manage stress and navigate setbacks.

Seek Professional Guidance:

Consult professionals like therapists, nutritionists, or trainers for personalized support and guidance.

Routine and Habit Formation:

Establish routines and habits for wellness that become ingrained in your daily life.

Self-Compassion:

Practice self-compassion by acknowledging that setbacks are a natural part of the journey. Treat yourself kindly and avoid self-criticism.

The Importance of Perseverance:

Perseverance is the ability to persist in your efforts despite challenges or difficulties. It plays a vital role in overcoming obstacles on your wellness journey:

Resilience:

Perseverance builds resilience, allowing you to bounce back from setbacks and continue forward.

Long-Term Success:

Wellness is a lifelong journey, and perseverance is the key to long-term success in maintaining healthy habits.

Personal Growth:

Overcoming obstacles fosters personal growth, as you learn to adapt, problem-solve, and develop resilience.

Achieving Goals:

Perseverance is the bridge between setting wellness goals and achieving them. It keeps you on course, even when faced with adversity.

Embracing Challenges:

Challenges are opportunities for growth and self-discovery. Embrace them with a mindset of perseverance.

Developing Perseverance:

Set Clear Intentions:

Clarify your intentions and motivations for your wellness journey. Having a strong why can fuel your perseverance.

Focus on Progress, Not Perfection:

Shift your focus from perfection to progress. Small steps and gradual improvements are worthy of celebration.

Positive Self-Talk:

Replace negative self-talk with positive and encouraging language. Self-belief is a powerful motivator.

Visualize Success:

Visualize yourself overcoming obstacles and achieving your wellness goals. Visualization can boost confidence and motivation.

Learn From Setbacks:

Approach setbacks as learning experiences. Analyze what went wrong and how you can adapt your approach.

Stay Connected:

Maintain connections with a supportive network of friends, family, or a wellness community. Shared experiences can provide motivation and encouragement.

Overcoming common obstacles requires perseverance, adaptability, and a growth mindset. By implementing these strategies and viewing challenges as opportunities for growth, you empower yourself to navigate obstacles and continue on your wellness journey.

Staying Motivated on Your Wellness Journey

Staying motivated on your wellness journey is essential for maintaining consistency and achieving your health and well-being goals. In this chapter, we will explore the importance of motivation, common sources of motivation, and strategies to sustain and reignite your motivation throughout your journey.

Understanding the Importance of Motivation:

Motivation serves as the driving force behind your wellness journey. It empowers you to:

Initiate Change:

Motivation inspires you to take the first steps toward adopting healthier habits and making positive changes in your life.

Maintain Consistency:

Motivation helps you stay committed to your wellness goals, even when faced with challenges or setbacks.

Overcome Obstacles:

When obstacles arise, motivation gives you the determination and resilience to find solutions and keep moving forward.

Celebrate Success:

Motivation fuels your sense of achievement and satisfaction when you reach milestones and accomplish your wellness objectives.

Common Sources of Motivation:

Intrinsic Motivation:

This comes from within and is driven by personal values, desires, and a genuine passion for your wellness journey.

Extrinsic Motivation:

External factors, such as rewards, recognition, or encouragement from others, can also motivate you.

Long-Term Goals:

The vision of long-term health and well-being can be a powerful motivator, driving you to make consistent choices that benefit your future self.

Short-Term Wins:

Celebrating small victories along the way can boost your motivation. These successes provide a sense of accomplishment and reinforce positive behaviors.

Accountability:

Sharing your goals with a friend, family member, or coach who holds you accountable can provide motivation through a sense of responsibility.

Strategies for Sustaining and Reigniting Motivation:

Set Clear and Specific Goals:

Clearly define your wellness goals, making them specific, measurable, achievable, relevant, and time-bound (SMART). Clarity enhances motivation.

Break Down Goals:

Divide long-term goals into smaller, manageable milestones. Achieving these milestones provides a sense of progress and motivation.

Visualize Success:

Regularly visualize yourself accomplishing your wellness goals. This mental imagery can boost your motivation and self-belief.

Create a Vision Board:

Construct a vision board featuring images, quotes, and reminders of your wellness goals. Display it where you can see it daily.

Celebrate Achievements:

Acknowledge and celebrate your successes, no matter how small they may seem. Rewarding yourself reinforces positive behavior.

Establish Routine:

Develop daily or weekly routines that incorporate wellness activities. Routines reduce decision fatigue and make it easier to stay on track.

Track Your Progress:

Keep a journal or use apps to track your progress. Recording your achievements can boost motivation.

Stay Informed:

Educate yourself about the benefits of wellness practices. Understanding how they impact your health can be motivating.

Seek Inspiration:

Read books, articles, or watch documentaries related to health and wellness. Exposure to inspiring stories and information can reignite motivation.

Find a Wellness Community:

Join or create a community of individuals with similar wellness goals. Sharing experiences and support can be highly motivating.

Mindfulness Practices:

Engage in mindfulness practices like meditation or deep breathing to reduce stress and stay present in your journey.

Adapt and Experiment:

Be open to adjusting your wellness routines and trying new approaches. Variety can prevent boredom and maintain motivation.

Reflect on Your "Why":

Regularly remind yourself of the reasons behind your wellness journey. Reconnecting with your motivations can reignite your commitment.

The Role of Resilience:

Maintaining motivation is closely linked to resilience—the ability to bounce back from setbacks and challenges. Cultivate resilience by viewing obstacles as opportunities for growth and learning.

Remember that motivation may ebb and flow, but with determination and the right strategies, you can reignite and sustain it on your wellness journey. Embrace the journey itself, celebrating each step forward, and keep your eyes on the long-term vision of a healthier and more fulfilling life.

9

Chapter 9

Preventive Health and Screening

Preventive health and regular screenings are fundamental components of your wellness journey, contributing to the early detection and prevention of health issues. In this chapter, we shall explore the significance of preventive health, the importance of regular screenings, and guidelines for maintaining optimal well-being through proactive healthcare.

Understanding the Importance of Preventive Health:

Preventive health encompasses a range of actions and practices designed to prevent the onset of health issues before they become more severe or difficult to manage. Key reasons for prioritizing preventive health include:

Early Detection: Preventive screenings can detect health problems at an early, more treatable stage, increasing the chances of successful intervention.

Cost-Effective: Preventive care is often more cost-effective than treating advanced health conditions, as it minimizes the need for expensive medical interventions.

Quality of Life: By addressing health concerns proactively, you can maintain or improve your quality of life and overall well-being.

Longevity: Prioritizing preventive health can contribute to a longer, healthier life, allowing you to enjoy more years of vitality and independence.

The Role of Regular Screenings:

Regular health screenings are an integral aspect of preventive health. These screenings involve the evaluation of specific health parameters to detect any deviations from normal values. Common screenings and their importance include:

Blood Pressure Monitoring:

Regular blood pressure checks help identify hypertension, a significant risk factor for heart disease and stroke.

Cholesterol Testing:

Monitoring cholesterol levels can detect elevated LDL ("bad") cholesterol, which is associated with cardiovascular disease.

Blood Sugar Tests:

Testing blood sugar levels can detect prediabetes or diabetes, a condition that can lead to various complications if left unmanaged.

Cancer Screenings:

Depending on your age and risk factors, cancer screenings such as mammograms, Pap smears, colonoscopies, and prostate-specific antigen (PSA) tests can detect cancer in its early stages.

Vaccinations:

Keeping up with recommended vaccinations helps prevent a range of infectious diseases, including flu, pneumonia, and certain types of cancer (e.g., HPV).

Bone Density Scans:

Bone density tests assess the risk of osteoporosis and fractures, helping to prevent bone-related issues.

Vision and Hearing Checks:

Regular eye and hearing exams can identify conditions like glaucoma, cataracts, and hearing loss.

Skin Checks:

Dermatological screenings can detect skin cancers, including melanoma.

Guidelines for Preventive Health:

Consult with Healthcare Providers:

Establish a relationship with primary care providers who can guide you on age-appropriate screenings and preventive measures.

Know Your Family History:

Be aware of your family's health history, as genetic factors can influence your risk of certain conditions.

Follow Guidelines:

Adhere to recommended screening guidelines based on your age, gender, and risk factors.

Healthy Lifestyle:

Maintain a healthy lifestyle through balanced nutrition, regular exercise, stress management, and adequate sleep.

Limit Risk Factors:

Minimize risk factors such as tobacco use, excessive alcohol consumption, and unsafe behaviors.

Stay Informed:

Stay informed about emerging health threats and recommendations, such as new vaccines or screenings.

Self-Examinations:

Learn and perform self-examinations as appropriate, such as breast or testicular self-exams.

Health Tracking:

Keep a record of your health history, including screenings, vaccinations, and any significant changes in your health.

Communicate Openly:

Share any health concerns or symptoms with your healthcare providers, even if they seem minor.

Regular Check-Ups:

Schedule regular check-ups with healthcare professionals to discuss your preventive health plan and address any concerns.

Preventive health and screenings are proactive measures to safeguard your well-being. By following recommended guidelines, maintaining a healthy lifestyle, and partnering with healthcare providers, you empower yourself to take control of your health and enjoy a longer, healthier life.

The Role of Preventive Care

The role of preventive care in your wellness journey cannot be overstated. It serves as the cornerstone of maintaining good health and proactively addressing potential health issues. In this chapter, we will delve into the critical role of preventive care, its benefits, and strategies to ensure you receive the right care at the right time.

Understanding the Role of Preventive Care:

Preventive care refers to healthcare services and measures aimed at preventing illness, detecting health conditions at an early stage, and promoting overall well-being. Its primary objectives are as follows:

Early Detection: Preventive care focuses on identifying health issues in their early, more treatable stages, which often leads to better outcomes.

Prevention: It emphasizes risk reduction and the prevention of health problems before they develop or worsen.

Quality of Life: By proactively addressing health concerns, preventive care helps you maintain or improve your quality of life.

Longevity: Prioritizing preventive care can contribute to a longer, healthier life, allowing you to enjoy more years of vitality.

The Benefits of Preventive Care:

Early Intervention: Preventive care identifies health issues before symptoms appear, allowing for prompt intervention and treatment.

Cost-Effective: Detecting and addressing health conditions early is often more cost-effective than treating advanced illnesses.

Improved Health: Regular preventive care can lead to better health outcomes and a reduced risk of complications.

Preventing Chronic Diseases: Many chronic diseases, such as diabetes, hypertension, and heart disease, can be managed or prevented through preventive measures.

Enhanced Well-Being: Prioritizing preventive care supports overall physical, mental, and emotional well-being.

Peace of Mind: Knowing that you're taking proactive steps to maintain your health can provide peace of mind and reduce anxiety about potential health issues.

Strategies for Effective Preventive Care:

Regular Check-Ups:

Schedule annual or biennial check-ups with your primary care provider. These appointments allow for a comprehensive assessment of your health.

Screenings:

Follow recommended screening guidelines based on your age, gender, and risk factors. These screenings may include blood pressure checks, cholesterol tests, mammograms, and more.

Vaccinations:

Stay up-to-date with recommended vaccinations to protect against infectious diseases.

Health Education:

Educate yourself about healthy lifestyle choices, nutrition, exercise, and stress management. Knowledge is a powerful tool for preventive care.

Family History:

Be aware of your family's health history, as it can influence your risk of certain conditions. Share this information with your healthcare provider.

Healthy Lifestyle:

Adopt a balanced diet, engage in regular physical activity, limit alcohol consumption, avoid tobacco use, and prioritize sleep.

Stress Management:

Practice stress-reduction techniques such as meditation, deep breathing, or yoga to support overall well-being.

Mental Health Care:

Prioritize your mental health by seeking help when needed. Mental well-being is an essential aspect of preventive care.

Self-Examinations:

Learn and perform self-examinations, such as breast or testicular self-exams, as appropriate for your age and gender.

Open Communication:

Maintain open and honest communication with your healthcare provider. Share any health concerns, symptoms, or changes in your health.

Preventive Medications:

If your healthcare provider recommends preventive medications, follow their advice and take prescribed medications as directed.

Regular Dental and Eye Exams:

Don't overlook dental and eye health. Regular dental check-ups and eye exams are essential components of preventive care.

Taking Control of Your Preventive Care:

Stay Informed:

Stay informed about recommended preventive care guidelines and updates. Knowledge empowers you to make informed decisions.

Set Reminders:

Use calendars, apps, or reminders to schedule and keep track of your preventive care appointments and screenings.

Advocate for Yourself:

Be an active advocate for your health. Ask questions, seek second opinions when necessary, and be proactive in your healthcare decisions.

Involve Your Healthcare Team:

Collaborate with your healthcare team to create a personalized preventive care plan tailored to your unique needs and risks.

Lifestyle Choices:

Embrace a healthy lifestyle, as your everyday choices have a profound impact on your preventive care efforts.

By recognizing the vital role of preventive care, adhering to recommended guidelines, and adopting a proactive approach to your health, you empower yourself to enjoy a life characterized by well-being, vitality, and longevity.

Health Screenings and Checkups

Health screenings and regular checkups are essential components of your wellness journey, serving as proactive measures to monitor your health, detect potential issues early, and ensure you receive appropriate care. In this chapter, we will delve into the importance of health screenings and checkups, recommended schedules, and guidelines to optimize these essential aspects of your well-being.

Understanding the Importance of Health Screenings and Checkups:

Health screenings and checkups are comprehensive evaluations of your physical and mental health. Their significance lies in:

Early Detection: Regular screenings can detect health conditions in their early stages, often before symptoms manifest, allowing for timely intervention and improved outcomes.

Preventive Care: These examinations are preventive measures that can identify risk factors and promote preventive strategies to reduce your likelihood of developing certain diseases.

Wellness Assessment: Health screenings and checkups provide a holistic assessment of your overall well-being, encompassing physical, mental, and emotional health.

Personalized Care: They allow healthcare providers to tailor recommendations and interventions based on your unique health profile and risk factors.

Recommended Health Screenings and Checkup Schedule:

The recommended schedule for health screenings and checkups can vary based on factors such as age, gender, family history, and individual health risks. Below is a general guideline:

Annual Checkups:

Physical Examination: An annual physical exam allows your healthcare provider to assess your general health, perform routine screenings, and address any concerns.

Blood Pressure Check: Monitor your blood pressure annually, or more frequently if you have hypertension or risk factors.

Biennial Checkups:

Cholesterol Testing: Starting in your 20s, consider cholesterol testing every 2 years, or as recommended by your healthcare provider.

Periodic Health Screenings:

Blood Sugar Testing: Depending on your risk factors, you may need blood sugar tests every 3 years or more frequently if you have diabetes risk factors.

Mammogram: Women should start mammogram screenings at age 40 and repeat them every 1-2 years, depending on individual risk factors and guidelines.

Pap Smear: Women should begin cervical cancer screenings with a Pap smear at age 21 and follow their healthcare provider's recommendations.

Colonoscopy: Starting at age 45 or earlier if you have risk factors, consider regular colonoscopies for colorectal cancer screening.

Prostate-Specific Antigen (PSA) Test: Men should discuss the need for PSA testing with their healthcare provider, considering their risk factors and age.

Bone Density Test: Women at or near menopause and those at risk for osteoporosis should discuss bone density testing with their healthcare provider.

Immunizations:

Stay up-to-date with recommended vaccinations throughout your life, including influenza, pneumonia, and others based on your age and health.

Dental and Eye Exams:

Schedule regular dental and eye exams as recommended by your dentist and eye care professional.

Guidelines for Optimal Health Screenings and Checkups:

Find a Trusted Healthcare Provider:

Establish a relationship with a healthcare provider who under-stands your medical history and can guide your preventive care.

Discuss Family History:

Share your family's health history with your healthcare provider, as it can influence your risk factors and screening recommendations.

Maintain Open Communication:

Discuss any health concerns or symptoms with your healthcare provider, even if they seem minor.

Adhere to Guidelines:

Follow recommended screening guidelines based on your age, gender, and risk factors. Be proactive in scheduling screenings.

Stay Informed:

Stay informed about the latest recommendations and guidelines for preventive care.

Record Keeping:

Maintain a record of your health screenings, test results, and immunizations for reference and easy access.

Lifestyle Choices:

Embrace a healthy lifestyle, as it significantly impacts your overall health and the effectiveness of preventive measures.

Mental Health Consideration:

Remember that mental health checkups and counseling can be just as important as physical health screenings for your overall well-being.

Health screenings and checkups are proactive steps you can take to safeguard your health and well-being. By following recommended guidelines, maintaining open communication with your healthcare provider, and prioritizing your preventive care, you empower yourself to enjoy a life characterized by optimal health and vitality.

Understanding Your Body's Signals

Understanding your body's signals is a fundamental aspect of your wellness journey. Your body communicates its needs, discomforts, and conditions through various signals and sensations. In this chapter, we will explore the importance of paying attention to these signals, how to interpret them, and the role they play in maintaining your overall health and well-being.

The Significance of Body Signals:

Your body is a remarkable and highly sophisticated system. It has an innate ability to provide feedback through signals and sensations. Understanding and responding to these signals is vital for several reasons:

Early Detection: Many health issues, when caught early, can be managed more effectively. Recognizing abnormal signals can lead to early intervention.

Preventive Care: Paying attention to your body's signals can help you make proactive choices that prevent health problems from developing in the first place.

Holistic Health: Body signals encompass physical, mental, and emotional sensations. Acknowledging these signals promotes holistic well-being.

Communication: Your body signals its needs, such as hunger or fatigue, which require your attention and response.

Common Body Signals and Their Interpretation:

Pain or Discomfort:

Pain is a clear signal that something is amiss. It can indicate injuries, inflammation, or underlying health conditions. It's essential to identify the location, type, and severity of pain and seek appropriate care.

Hunger and Thirst:

Hunger and thirst signals are your body's way of telling you it needs nourishment or hydration. Listen to these signals to maintain energy levels and overall health.

Fatigue:

Fatigue signals the need for rest and recovery. Ignoring this signal can lead to burnout and decreased productivity. Adequate sleep and breaks are crucial.

Emotional Signals:

Emotions like stress, anxiety, sadness, and joy are signals from your mind and heart. Acknowledging and managing emotions is essential for mental and emotional well-being.

Nausea or Digestive Discomfort:

These signals can indicate issues with your digestive system or food intolerances. Identifying trigger foods and seeking medical advice if problems persist is crucial.

Changes in Skin and Appearance:

Skin changes, such as rashes, acne, or unusual moles, may signal skin conditions or other health concerns. Regular skin checks are important.

Temperature and Sensations:

Feeling too hot or cold can indicate temperature-related discomfort or underlying conditions. Adjusting your environment accordingly is important.

Changes in Sleep Patterns:

Insomnia, excessive sleepiness, or changes in sleep quality may signal stress, medical conditions, or sleep disorders.

Changes in Urination and Bowel Movements:

Variations in urination frequency, color, or consistency of bowel movements can signal underlying digestive or urinary issues.

Strategies for Understanding and Responding to Body Signals:

Mindfulness: Cultivate mindfulness to become more aware of your body's signals. Mindfulness practices like meditation can help you tune in to your body.

Keep a Health Journal: Maintain a journal to record any recurring or unusual body signals, along with relevant details like timing, severity, and associated factors.

Consult Healthcare Providers: If you experience persistent or concerning signals, consult healthcare professionals for assessment and guidance.

Lifestyle Adjustments: Address signals by making appropriate lifestyle changes, such as adjusting your diet, exercise routine, sleep patterns, or stress management techniques.

Seek Mental Health Support: If emotional signals persist or impact your daily life, consider seeking support from a mental health professional.

Regular Health Checkups: Schedule regular checkups with your healthcare provider to discuss any body signals, even if they seem minor.

Trust Your Intuition: Listen to your gut feelings or intuition. If something feels off, it's worth investigating.

Understanding and responding to your body's signals is a proactive and empowering approach to maintaining your health and well-being. By recognizing and respecting these signals, you can address issues early, prevent potential problems, and support your body in its quest for balance and vitality.

10

Chapter 10

Long-Term Wellness and Aging

Long-term wellness and aging are intimately connected aspects of your wellness journey. Aging is a natural and inevitable process, but the choices you make throughout your life profoundly influence your well-being as you age. In this chapter, we will explore the concepts of long-term wellness and aging gracefully, providing insights and strategies to support your health and vitality as you grow older.

Embracing Long-Term Wellness:

Long-term wellness encompasses maintaining good health, vitality, and a high quality of life throughout the aging process. It involves nurturing physical, mental, and emotional well-being with the understanding that wellness is a lifelong journey. Key elements of long-term wellness include:

Lifestyle Choices: The habits you cultivate, such as nutrition, exercise, sleep, and stress management, play a significant role in your long-term wellness.

Preventive Care: Regular checkups, health screenings, and preventive measures help identify and address health issues early.

Mental and Emotional Health: Nurturing mental and emotional well-being is essential for long-term wellness. This includes managing stress, seeking support when needed, and practicing mindfulness.

Healthy Relationships: Social connections and supportive relationships contribute to overall well-being, especially in later years.

Positive Aging Attitude: Embrace aging as a natural part of life and focus on the opportunities and wisdom that come with it.

Strategies for Long-Term Wellness:

Healthy Lifestyle: Maintain a balanced diet, engage in regular physical activity, prioritize sleep, and manage stress throughout your life.

Mental and Emotional Well-Being: Develop emotional resilience, practice mindfulness, and seek support for mental health when necessary.

Regular Health Checkups: Schedule regular health checkups to monitor your health, discuss preventive care, and address any concerns.

Stay Active: Engage in physical activities that suit your age and abilities. Regular exercise promotes strength, flexibility, and cardiovascular health.

Nutrition: Focus on a diet rich in fruits, vegetables, whole grains, lean proteins, and healthy fats. Adequate hydration is also crucial.

Social Connections: Foster and maintain social connections with family, friends, and your community to combat loneliness and isolation.

Cognitive Stimulation: Keep your mind active through life-long learning, puzzles, reading, or engaging in intellectually stimulating activities.

Quality Sleep: Prioritize good sleep hygiene to ensure restorative sleep, as sleep quality is closely linked to overall well-being.

Positive Attitude: Cultivate a positive attitude toward aging. Embrace the wisdom and experience that come with getting older.

Aging Gracefully:

Aging gracefully is about approaching the aging process with acceptance, optimism, and a focus on well-being. It involves:

Self-Care: Continue prioritizing self-care and well-being throughout your life, adapting your routines as needed.

Adaptation: Be open to adapting your lifestyle and routines to accommodate changing needs and abilities as you age.

Mental Agility: Challenge your mind with new experiences and learning opportunities to maintain mental agility.

Acceptance: Embrace the changes that come with aging, recognizing that they are a natural part of life.

Seeking Support: If you encounter health challenges, seek appropriate support and medical care.

Enjoying Life: Continue to pursue your passions, hobbies, and interests, finding joy and fulfillment in each stage of life.

The Importance of Planning:

While embracing long-term wellness and aging gracefully is vital, it's also essential to plan for your future. Consider aspects such as financial security, healthcare, and end-of-life wishes. Planning ahead can provide peace of mind and ensure your well-being is supported in later years.

Long-term wellness and aging are interconnected aspects of your wellness journey. By making informed choices, maintaining a healthy lifestyle, nurturing mental and emotional well-being, and embracing the aging process with positivity and resilience, you empower yourself to age gracefully while enjoying a high quality of life.

Wellness Across the Lifespan

Wellness across the lifespan is a multifaceted journey that evolves with each stage of life. Your well-being is influenced by a combination of biological, psychological, social, and environmental factors, and understanding how these factors intersect at different ages is essential for lifelong health and vitality. In this chapter, we will explore wellness considerations at various stages of life, from infancy to old age, providing insights and strategies to support your well-being throughout your journey.

Wellness in Infancy and Childhood:

Nutrition: Infants and children require proper nutrition for growth and development. Breastfeeding, a balanced diet, and regular pediatric checkups are essential.

Physical Activity: Encourage physical activity through play and exploration to develop motor skills and promote a healthy lifestyle from an early age.

Mental Development: Support cognitive development through interactive play, reading, and exposure to a variety of experiences.

Emotional Well-Being: Create a nurturing and supportive environment to foster emotional well-being, as early experiences significantly impact mental health.

Wellness in Adolescence:

Healthy Habits: Adolescents should develop healthy habits related to nutrition, physical activity, and sleep to support growth and prevent future health issues.

Mental Health: Address the unique emotional and psychological challenges of adolescence through open communication and access to mental health support.

Social Connections: Encourage healthy social relationships, as peer interactions play a crucial role in emotional development.

Wellness in Adulthood:

Healthy Lifestyle: Maintain a balanced diet, regular exercise, and stress management to support overall well-being.

Career and Relationships: Focus on career development and the cultivation of meaningful relationships, as these contribute to mental and emotional wellness.

Family Planning: Consider family planning and reproductive health decisions, ensuring they align with your life goals and values.

Wellness in Middle Age:

Physical Health: Prioritize regular health screenings and preventive care as age-related health concerns may arise.

Mental and Emotional Health: Manage stress, nurture emotional well-being, and seek support when facing life transitions.

Maintain Social Connections: Sustain and strengthen social networks, as maintaining relationships becomes increasingly important.

Career and Financial Planning: Reevaluate career goals and financial plans to prepare for retirement and future well-being.

Wellness in Older Age:

Healthcare: Continue to prioritize regular checkups, screenings, and preventive care to address age-related health concerns.

Mental Agility: Engage in activities that stimulate mental agility, such as puzzles, learning, and cognitive exercises.

Physical Activity: Maintain physical activity to promote mobility and overall health, adjusting routines as necessary.

Social Engagement: Stay socially active to combat isolation and maintain a sense of purpose and community.

End-of-Life Planning: Consider end-of-life wishes, including healthcare directives and financial planning, to ensure your well-being in later years.

Wellness across the lifespan is a dynamic and evolving journey, with each stage presenting unique challenges and opportunities. By recognizing the importance of nurturing physical, mental, and emotional well-being at different ages and adapting your lifestyle accordingly, you can enjoy a life characterized by health, vitality, and fulfillment.

Healthy Aging Strategies

Healthy aging is a lifelong endeavor that involves nurturing physical, mental, and emotional well-being as you grow older. It's about embracing the aging process with vitality, purpose, and a focus on maintaining a high quality of life. In this chapter, we will delve into strategies for healthy aging, providing insights and guidelines to support your well-being in later years.

Physical Well-Being:

Nutrition: Maintain a balanced diet rich in fruits, vegetables, whole grains, lean proteins, and healthy fats. Adequate hydration is crucial for overall health.

Regular Exercise: Engage in regular physical activity that suits your age and abilities. Include cardiovascular, strength, flexibility, and balance exercises to support mobility and prevent age-related issues.

Bone Health: Incorporate calcium and vitamin D-rich foods into your diet to support bone health. Weight-bearing exercises are also essential.

Regular Check-Ups: Schedule regular check-ups with your healthcare provider to monitor your health, discuss preventive care, and address any age-related concerns.

Medication Management: If prescribed medications, adhere to your healthcare provider's instructions and discuss any side effects or concerns.

Mental and Emotional Well-Being:

Stimulate Your Mind: Engage in mentally stimulating activities such as reading, puzzles, learning a new skill, or pursuing hobbies that challenge your cognitive abilities.

Social Engagement: Stay socially active by maintaining relationships with friends, family, and your community. Social connections are vital for mental and emotional health.

Manage Stress: Practice stress-reduction techniques like meditation, deep breathing, or yoga to manage the impact of stress on your well-being.

Seek Support: If you experience mental health challenges, such as depression or anxiety, seek professional support and counseling.

Lifestyle Choices:

Tobacco and Alcohol: Avoid tobacco use, and limit alcohol consumption to moderate levels or as recommended by your healthcare provider.

Sleep Quality: Prioritize good sleep hygiene to ensure restorative sleep, as sleep quality is closely linked to overall well-being.

Safety: Make necessary safety adaptations in your home to prevent falls and injuries, especially if mobility or balance is a concern.

Positive Aging Attitude:

Mindset: Embrace aging as a natural part of life and focus on the opportunities and wisdom that come with it.

Purpose: Cultivate a sense of purpose and engagement in meaningful activities that bring joy and fulfillment.

Adaptation: Be open to adapting your lifestyle and routines to accommodate changing needs and abilities as you age.

Preventive Care:

Regular Health Screenings: Continue to prioritize regular health screenings and preventive care to address age-related health concerns.

Immunizations: Stay up-to-date with recommended vaccinations, including flu and pneumonia vaccines.

End-of-Life Planning: Consider end-of-life wishes, including healthcare directives and financial planning, to ensure your well-being in later years and provide peace of mind.

Social Connections:

Community Involvement: Participate in community activities, volunteer work, or clubs to stay socially engaged.

Family and Friends: Maintain and strengthen your relationships with family and friends, as social connections remain important for overall well-being.

Healthy aging is an attainable goal that requires a proactive and holistic approach. By nurturing your physical, mental, and emotional well-being, embracing a positive attitude toward aging, and seeking support when needed, you empower yourself to age gracefully while enjoying a life characterized by vitality and fulfillment.

Preparing for a Bright Future

Preparing for a bright future is a journey marked by intentional choices, continued growth, and a focus on creating a life filled with purpose, fulfillment, and well-being. In this chapter, we will explore strategies and considerations to help you shape a future that aligns with your aspirations, values, and vision for a fulfilling life.

Defining Your Vision:

Reflect on Your Goals: Take time to reflect on your short-term and long-term goals. Consider what you want to achieve in various aspects of your life, including career, relationships, and personal development.

Clarify Your Values: Identify your core values and principles. Understanding what truly matters to you will guide your decisions and help you create a future that aligns with your values.

Educational and Career Development:

Lifelong Learning: Embrace a mindset of lifelong learning. Seek opportunities for continued education, skill development, and personal growth.

Career Planning: Set clear career goals and develop a plan to achieve them. This may involve pursuing further education, seeking mentorship, or exploring new career paths.

Networking: Cultivate a professional network by connecting with colleagues, mentors, and industry peers. Networking can open doors to new opportunities and collaborations.

Financial Well-Being:

Financial Planning: Create a comprehensive financial plan that includes savings, investments, and retirement planning. Consult with financial experts to ensure your financial well-being.

Budgeting: Practice responsible budgeting to manage your finances effectively and save for your future goals.

Health and Wellness:

Health Maintenance: Prioritize your physical and mental health through regular check-ups, preventive care, and healthy lifestyle choices.

Wellness Practices: Incorporate wellness practices into your daily routine, such as exercise, stress management, and mindfulness, to promote overall well-being.

Relationships and Community:

Nurturing Relationships: Cultivate and maintain meaningful relationships with family, friends, and your community. Social connections play a significant role in well-being.

Community Involvement: Get involved in your community through volunteer work or engagement in causes that matter to you. Giving back can be a fulfilling aspect of your future.

Personal Growth and Fulfillment:

Setting Boundaries: Learn to set healthy boundaries to protect your time, energy, and well-being.

Self-Care: Prioritize self-care practices that rejuvenate your mind, body, and spirit.

Pursue Passions: Dedicate time to pursuing your passions and hobbies, as they bring joy and fulfillment to your life.

Embracing Change:

Adaptability: Cultivate adaptability and resilience to navigate life's inevitable changes and challenges.

Open-Mindedness: Remain open to new experiences, perspectives, and opportunities that may enrich your future.

End-of-Life Planning:

Legal and Financial Documents: Ensure that your legal and financial affairs, such as wills, advance directives, and power of attorney, are in order.

Discuss Your Wishes: Communicate your end-of-life wishes with loved ones to provide clarity and ensure your desires are respected.

Preparing for a bright future is a continuous process that involves setting goals, making intentional choices, and nurturing your well-being across various life domains. By defining your vision, pursuing educational and career development, maintaining financial well-being, prioritizing health and wellness, fostering relationships, and embracing personal growth, you empower yourself to shape a future filled with purpose, fulfillment, and opportunities for growth.

Celebrating Your Progress

Celebrating your progress is a vital aspect of your wellness journey. Acknowledging your achievements, no matter how small, provides motivation, reinforces positive habits, and fosters a sense of accomplishment. In this chapter, we will explore the importance of celebrating your progress and offer strategies for doing so effectively.

Why Celebrate Your Progress:

Motivation: Celebrating your achievements provides motivation to continue working toward your goals. It reinforces the idea that your efforts are paying off.

Positive Reinforcement: Acknowledging your progress reinforces positive habits and behaviors, making them more likely to become ingrained in your daily life.

Boosting Confidence: Celebrating your achievements boosts your self-confidence and self-esteem, empowering you to take on new challenges.

Recognizing Effort: It's essential to recognize the effort you put into your wellness journey, even if you haven't yet reached your ultimate goals.

Strategies for Celebrating Your Progress:

Set Milestones: Break your long-term goals into smaller, achievable milestones. Celebrate each milestone as you reach it.

Reward Yourself: Treat yourself to a reward when you achieve a significant milestone. This could be a small indulgence, a favorite activity, or something special you've been wanting.

Share Your Achievements: Share your progress with a trusted friend, family member, or support group. Sharing your successes with others can make the celebration more meaningful.

Journal Your Successes: Keep a journal or progress diary where you record your achievements, no matter how minor they may seem. Reflect on how far you've come.

Visual Reminders: Create visual reminders of your progress. This could be a vision board, a chart, or a collection of photos that represent your achievements.

Practice Gratitude: Take a moment to express gratitude for the progress you've made. Gratitude can enhance your sense of well-being.

Celebrate Health Milestones: Celebrate improvements in your health, such as achieving a healthy weight, reaching fitness milestones, or hitting specific wellness targets.

Reflect on Positive Changes: Reflect on the positive changes you've made in your life as a result of your wellness journey. This could include improved relationships, increased energy, or reduced stress.

Set New Goals: After celebrating your progress, set new goals to continue your journey of growth and improvement.

Celebrate Others: Celebrate the achievements of others in your support network. Recognizing their progress can strengthen your sense of community and mutual support.

Mindset Matters:

Focus on the Journey: Emphasize the importance of the journey itself, not just the destination. Celebrating small wins along the way enhances the overall experience.

Practice Self-Compassion: Be kind to yourself, especially when faced with setbacks or challenges. Self-compassion encourages resilience and perseverance.

Learn from Setbacks: Instead of dwelling on setbacks, view them as opportunities for growth and learning. Celebrate your resilience in the face of adversity.

Celebrating your progress is a meaningful and essential part of your wellness journey. By setting milestones, rewarding yourself, sharing your achievements, and maintaining a positive mindset, you not only acknowledge your accomplishments but also fuel your motivation to continue working toward your goals. Remember that celebrating progress is a way to honor the effort you invest in your well-being and to embrace the journey of self-improvement.

Resources for Further Exploration

As you embark on your wellness journey, it's essential to have access to a wealth of resources and information to support your growth and well-being. In this chapter, I will provide a comprehensive list of resources for further exploration, covering various aspects of wellness, including physical health, mental well-being, personal development, and more.

Books on Wellness and Health:

"The Blue Zones: Lessons for Living Longer From the People Who've Lived the Longest" by Dan Buettner

"The Power of Habit: Why We Do What We Do in Life and Business" by Charles Duhigg

"Atomic Habits: An Easy & Proven Way to Build Good Habits & Break Bad Ones" by James Clear

"The Whole-Body Microbiome: How to Harness Microbes—Inside and Out—for Lifelong Health" by B. Brett Finlay and Jessica M. Finlay

"Why We Sleep: Unlocking the Power of Sleep and Dreams" by Matthew Walker

Mental Health Resources:

National Alliance on Mental Illness (NAMI): **www.nami.org**

American Psychological Association (APA): **www.apa.org**

Mental Health America (MHA): **www.mhanational.org**

Headspace - Meditation and Mindfulness App: **www.headspace.com**

Physical Health and Nutrition:

American Heart Association: **www.heart.org**

Centers for Disease Control and Prevention (CDC): **www.cdc.gov**

MyPlate by USDA - Nutrition Guidelines: **www.choosemy-plate.gov**

Mayo Clinic - Health Information: **www.mayoclinic.org**

Fitness and Exercise:

American Council on Exercise (ACE): **www.acefitness.org**

Bodybuilding.com - Exercise and Nutrition: **www.bodybuilding.com**

CrossFit – Fitness Community: **www.crossfit.com**

Lifestyle and Personal Development:

TED Talks - Inspiring Talks on Various Topics: **www.ted.com**

The Art of Manliness - Personal Development and Lifestyle: **www.artofmanliness.com**

Zen Habits - Minimalism and Simple Living: **zenhabits.net**

Mindfulness and Meditation:

Insight Timer – Meditation App: **www.insighttimer.com**

Calm - Meditation and Sleep App: **www.calm.com**

Mindful.org – Resources for Mindfulness Practice: **www.mindful.org**

Nutrition and Recipe Websites:

AllRecipes – Healthy Recipe Ideas: **www.allrecipes.com**

EatingWell – Nutrition and Healthy Cooking: **www.eating-well.com**

Minimalist Baker – Simple and Healthy Recipes: **minimalist-baker.com**

Exercise Apps:

Nike Training Club – Fitness App: **www.nike.com/ntc-app**

Strava – Running and Cycling App: **www.strava.com**

MyFitnessPal – Fitness and Nutrition Tracker: **www.myfitness-pal.com**

Wellness Podcasts:

"The Tony Robbins Podcast" – Personal Development: **www.tonyrobbins.com/podcast**

"The School of Greatness" with Lewis Howes – Inspiration and Growth: **www.lewishowes.com/blog**

Financial Well-Being:

Dave Ramsey – Personal Finance and Budgeting: **www.daver-amsey.com**

The Motley Fool – Investing and Financial Advice: **www.fool.com**

Mindfulness and Meditation Resources

Mindfulness and meditation are powerful practices for enhancing your mental and emotional well-being, reducing stress, and fostering inner peace. In this chapter, I will provide a curated list of mindfulness and meditation resources to support your journey towards a more mindful and centered life.

Mindfulness Apps and Websites:

Headspace: A widely popular mindfulness app offering guided meditation sessions, sleep stories, and mindfulness exercises. **Website**

Calm: Known for its soothing meditations, sleep stories, and relaxation exercises, Calm is a go-to app for stress reduction. **Website**

Insight Timer: A meditation app with a vast library of guided meditations, talks, and courses led by meditation teachers from around the world. **Website**

Mindful.org: An online resource dedicated to mindfulness and meditation, offering articles, guided practices, and expert insights. **Website**

UCLA Mindful Awareness Research Center (MARC): Provides free guided meditations and mindfulness resources developed by mindfulness experts. **Website**

Books on Mindfulness and Meditation:

"The Miracle of Mindfulness" by Thich Nhat Hanh: A classic book on mindfulness by the renowned Zen master Thich Nhat Hanh.

"Wherever You Go, There You Are" by Jon Kabat-Zinn: A guide to mindfulness meditation by the creator of the Mindfulness-Based Stress Reduction (MBSR) program.

"Radical Acceptance" by Tara Brach: A transformative book exploring self-compassion and mindfulness.

"The Untethered Soul" by Michael A. Singer: Explores the concept of mindfulness and inner peace through profound insights.